Lecture Notes in Computer Science 8331

Commenced Publication in 1973
Founding and Former Series Editors:
Gerhard Goos, Juris Hartmanis, and Jan van Leeuwen

For further volumes:
http://www.springer.com/series/7412

Bjoern Menze · Georg Langs
Albert Montillo · Michael Kelm
Henning Müller · Zhuowen Tu (Eds.)

Medical
Computer Vision

Large Data in Medical Imaging

Third International MICCAI Workshop, MCV 2013
Nagoya, Japan, September 26, 2013
Revised Selected Papers

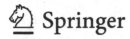
Springer

Editors

Bjoern Menze
ETH
Zürich
Switzerland

and

Technical University of Munich
Munich
Germany

Georg Langs
Medical University of Vienna
Vienna
Austria

Albert Montillo
GE Global Research
Niskayuna, NY
USA

Michael Kelm
Siemens AG
Erlangen
Germany

Henning Müller
University of Applied Sciences
    Western Switzerland
Sierre
Switzerland

Zhuowen Tu
University of California
La Jolla, CA
USA

ISSN 0302-9743   ISSN 1611-3349 (electronic)
ISBN 978-3-319-05529-9   ISBN 978-3-319-05530-5 (eBook)
DOI 10.1007/978-3-319-05530-5
Springer Cham Heidelberg New York Dordrecht London

Library of Congress Control Number: 2014934685

LNCS Sublibrary: SL6 – Image Processing, Computer Vision, Pattern Recognition, and Graphics

Printed on acid-free paper

Springer is part of Springer Science+Business Media (www.springer.com)

Preface

This book includes articles from the 2013 MICCAI (Medical Image Computing for Computer-Assisted Intervention) workshop on Medical Computer Vision (MCV) that was held on September 26, 2013, in Nagoya, Japan. The workshop followed up on similar events in the past years held in conjunction with MICCAI and CVPR.

The workshop received 25 high-quality submissions that were all reviewed by at least three external reviewers. Borderline papers were further reviewed by the organizers to obtain the most objective decisions for the final paper selection. Seven papers (28%) were accepted as oral presentations and another 12 (48%) as posters including a short presentation. The review process was double blind.

In addition to the accepted oral presentations and posters, the workshop had two invited speakers. Leo Grady of HeartFlow Inc., USA, discussed the challenge of employing segmentation routines in real clinical settings, addressing the problem of cardiac CT analysis. He stressed that segmentation routines should not remain in academic settings but should be evaluated for their impact in real applications, as small differences in the segmentation can sometimes lead to totally differing decisions. Then, Ron Kikinis of Harvard Medical School presented an overview of the development of the medical imaging community. He used the 3D Slicer software as an example and showed how the impact of methods increases when they can easily be modified by other researchers.

The award for the best paper was sponsored by Siemens Corporate Technology. It was given to Stefan Bauer et al., who presented the paper "Integrated Spatio-temporal Segmentation of Longitudinal Brain Tumour Imaging Studies." In particular the longitudinal nature of the analysis and the detailed evaluation of the automatic segmentation over time were considered important.

In general, the workshop resulted in many lively discussions and showed well the current trends and tendencies in medical computer vision and how the techniques can be used in clinical work. These proceedings start with a short overview of the topics that were discussed during the workshop as well as the discussions that took place during the sessions, followed by the 19 accepted papers of the workshop and two invited and reviewed papers that were presented in the "VISCERAL Challenge Session" – describing the segmentation task and data set of the VISCERAL benchmark challenge.

We would like to thank all the reviewers who helped in selecting high-quality papers for the workshop and the authors for submitting and presenting high-quality research all of which made MICCAI-MCV 2013 a great success. We plan to organize a similar workshop in next year's MICCAI conference in Boston.

November 2013

Bjoern Menze
Georg Langs
Albert Montillo
Michael Kelm
Henning Müller
Zhuowen Tu

Organization

Organizing Committee

General Co-chairs

Bjoern Menze   Switzerland
Georg Langs   Austria
Albert Montillo   USA
Michael Kelm   Germany
Henning Müller   Switzerland
Zhuowen Tu   USA

Publication Chair

Henning Müller   Switzerland

International Program Committee

Tal Arbel   McGill University, Canada
Horst Bischof   TU Graz, Austria
Marleen de Bruijne   Erasmus MC Rotterdam, The Netherlands
Dirk Breitenreicher   Google, USA
Philippe Cattin   University of Basel, Switzerland
Ertan Cetingul   Siemens Corporate Research, USA
Antonio Criminisi   Microsoft Research Cambridge, UK
Adrien Depeursinge   Stanford, USA
Marius Erdt   Fraunhofer/NTU, Singapore
Jurgen Gall   Max Planck Institute, Tübingen, Germany
Tobias Gass   ETH Zurich, Switzerland
Alwina Goh   National University, Singapore
Allan Hanbury   TU Vienna, Austria
Juan Eugenio Iglesias   Harvard Medical School, USA
Ron Kikinis   Harvard Medical School, USA
Ender Konukoglu   Harvard Medical School, USA
Herve Lombaert   McGill University, Canada
Xinghua Lou   Memorial Sloan-Kettering Cancer Center New York, USA
Le Lu   NIH, USA
Jan Margeta   Inria, France
Diana Mateus   TU Munich, Germany
Nassir Navab   TU Munich, Germany
Marc Niethammer   UNC Chapel Hill, USA

Sponsors

European Commission 7th Framework Programme, VISCERAL (318068) and Siemens AG, Corporate Technology for the best paper prize.

Contents

Detection and Localization

Features and Retrieval

VISCERAL Session

Workshop Overview

Overview of the 2013 Workshop on Medical Computer Vision (MCV 2013)

Henning Müller[1,2](✉), Bjoern H. Menze[3,4], Georg Langs[5,6], Albert Montillo[7],
B. Michael Kelm[8], Zhuowen Tu[9], and Óscar Alfonso Jiménez del Toro[1]

[1] University of Applied Sciences Western Switzerland (HES–SO), Sierre, Switzerland
henning.mueller@hevs.ch
[2] University Hospitals and University of Geneva, Geneva, Switzerland
[3] ETHZ Zürich, Zürich, Switzerland
[4] INRIA, Sophia–Antipolis, France
[5] Medical University of Vienna, Wien, Austria
[6] MIT, Cambridge, MA, USA
[7] GE Global Research, Niskayuna, NY, USA
[8] Imaging and Computer Vision, Siemens AG, Corporate Technology,
Erlangen, Germany
[9] UCLA, Los Angeles, CA, USA

Abstract. The 2013 workshop in medical computer vision (MCV) took
place in Nagoya, Japan in connection with MICCAI (Medical Image
Computing for Computer Assisted Intervention). It is the third MICCAI
MCV workshop after 2011 and 2012 also related to a similar workshop
held at CVPR (Computer Vision and Pattern Recognition) in 2012. The
workshop aims at exploring the use of modern computer vision technology in tasks such as automatic segmentation and registration, localisation of anatomical features and detection of anomalies. It emphasises
questions of harvesting, organising and learning from large–scale medical imaging data sets and general–purpose automatic understanding of
medical images. We are especially interested in modern, scalable and efficient algorithms which generalise well to previously unseen images. The
strong participation of over 70 persons in the workshop shows the importance and timeliness of medical computer vision as a research field. This
overview article describes the papers presented in the workshop as either
oral presentations or short presentations and posters. It also describes the
invited talks and the results of the VISCERAL session in the workshop
on the use of big data in medical imaging.

Keywords: Medical image analysis · Medical computer vision · Segmentation · Detection

1 Introduction

The workshop MCV (Medical Computer Vision) took place in connection with
the MICCAI (Medical Image Computing for Computer–Assisted Interventions)

B. Menze et al. (Eds.): MCV 2013, LNCS 8331, pp. 3–10, 2014.
DOI: 10.1007/978-3-319-05530-5_1, © Springer International Publishing Switzerland 2014

Conference on September 26, 2013 in Nagoya, Japan. It was the third workshop on medical computer vision organised in connection with MICCAI after the workshops in 2010 [18] and 2012 [17]. The workshop received 25 high quality paper submissions. All papers were reviewed by at least three external reviewers of the scientific committee of the workshop. Then, all borderline papers were reviewed in addition by at least one workshop organisers. The seven best papers were presented as long papers and another twelve papers were accepted as short papers and posters.

Triggered by the increasing importance of large datasets it was decided to add a session on an evaluation campaign called VISCERAL[1] (VISual Concept ExtRaction challenge in RAdioLogy) in 2013. The VISCERAL project [15] is funded by the EU, and aims at making a substantial body of annotated medical imaging data available to the community. VISCERAL will conduct two benchmarking campaigns to create a comprehensive state of the art in medical computer vision aiming at localization, segmentation and retrieval in medical imaging data. The first batch of manually annotated 3D medical data for the first benchmark was distributed before the workshop. The first benchmark focusses on the automatic detection and segmentation of organs in the body and includes over 20 organs and more than 20 landmarks in the body. The second benchmark will focus on the retrieval of similar cases in very large data sets. Two papers in this volume present preliminary work on the VISCERAL data set and the discussion at the workshop on the important parts of the benchmark and the challenges.

The workshop attracted more than 70 participants, which provided ample opportunity for very interesting discussions during the workshop and also during the coffee and lunch breaks. The topics ranged from the application of concepts such as classification or regression in novel contexts, to the realistic evaluation of methods in the context of big data.

This text provides an overview of the most important discussions that took place during the medical computer vision workshop and the challenges that were identified in the field.

2   Papers Presented at the Workshop

The workshop presents several categories of papers that are described in more detail in the following sections. *Long papers* include the papers with the best review scores that were presented orally at the MCV workshop. The *short papers* were high quality papers accepted for a short oral presentation at the workshop and a poster. Then, the two *invited talks* are described. The last section finally describes the VISCERAL session of the workshop and the two preliminary papers that were presented by participants in the organ detection challenge. This section also describes the discussions during the VISCERAL session.

---

[1] http://visceral.eu/

2.1   Long Papers

The presented long papers were separated into three topic areas, papers on registration techniques, segmentations techniques and a last section on localisation and detection.

Registration. Chen-Rui Chou et al. describe a 2D/3D deformable registration approach based on first assigning an image a certain partion of the training example set, and then applying a projection matrix based on linear regression [4]. John Onofrey then demonstrated that semi-supervised learning can improve image registration [19] significantly.

Segmentation. Ryan Cabeen et al. proposed a clustering based method to generate supervoxels in diffusion MR imaging data of the white matter [3]. Stefan Bauer et al. won the best paper prize sponsored by Siemens Corporate Technology for their contribution on integrated fully automatic spatio–temporal segmentation of longitudinal brain tumor imaging studies highly relevant for disease grading [2]. Quan Wang et al. proposed a two stage approach to segment knee cartilage that uses the relative position to the bone [22].

Detection and Localization. Kiryl Chykeyuk and Alison Noble demonstrated how class-specific regression random forests can be use to extract standard planes from 3D echocardiography data [5]. Then, Qi Song et al., proposed hierarchical active appearance models working on automatically detected landmark candidates in pairs of anterior-posterior and lateral view radiographs [20].

2.2   Short Papers

The short papers are grouped into the topics of Detection, Visualization, Segmentation and Features and Retrieval in the following subsections.

Detection. Ghesu et al. propose in [11] a new approach to detect the pectoral muscle in digital breast tomosynthesis and mammography for breast cancer screening and diagnosis obtaining better results on a group of 95 patients than traditional approaches. This paper was runner up for the best paper award of the workshop. In [24], Zheng et al. detect and track the aorta in non–contrast enhanced images using the Hough transform. Fully automatic aorta segmentation can be useful for a variety of applications. Domingos et al. work on 3D ultrasound images in [7] .The approach detects left vendtrical apical views using a mix between a model–based approach and a machine–learning–based approach.

Visualization. German Corredor et al. propose in [6] an architecture for flexible visualisation of microscopy images at several levels. Microscopy images can be extremely large in size and new models ae required for efficiently viewing them. The approach presented improve over the stander JPEG2000 model that is commonly used. Again another imaging modality is used in [1]. Aly Abdelrehim et al. try constructing 3D models of teeth based on singe images. A 2D PCA approach is used to improve the reconstruction quality over the current state of the art.

Segmentation. Alfiia Galimzianova et al. [10] describe an unsupervised approach for segmentation of brain MR images. A robust mixture–parameter estimation is proposed that detects outliers as samples with low significance, leading to better results than standard techniques. Also in [23] an approach for brain segmentation is presented, this time for Alzheimer patients using an atlas–based approach and targeting several structures of the brain. The algorithm was tested on several Alzheimer patients and healthy controls.

Features and Retrieval. In [16], Le Lu et al. propose a multi–level feature learning approach for computer aided diagnosis. The approach learns features on a voxel–, instance– and database–level and is applied to different types of lung nodules in CT images. An interesting approach to map features from 2D images and 3D images into a single feature space is proposed in [13] using singular value decomposition. This allows to search with 2D image examples for visually similar 3D volumes. A novel shape descriptor for classifying polyps in colonoscopy images is proposed in [12]. It uses several shape descriptors on the polyp blobs. The articles also analyses the influence of image enhancement on the performance of the features. In both [8] and [9] celiac disease is targeted. The first articles describes a shape feature for better diagnosis, that is of good quality and gives a very compact description. In the second text, Gadermayr et al. describe a method that allows to compute features from the endoscopy images without the usual requirement of distortion correction, which is directly integrated into the feature extractor and removes the problems linked to image rasterisation. This paper was a runner up for the best paper award at the workshop.

2.3   Invited Papers

The first invited speaker was *Leo Grady* of Healthflow Inc., USA. Leo Grady is active in both the medical imaging and the computer vision communities, and is currently focussing his research efforts on highly accurate segmentation in 3D data. His invited talk focused on the remaining challenges in image segmentation for real clinical applications. The non-invasive assessment of coronary artery disease is a central basis for treatment decisions that can range from surgery to medication. Small differences in the segmentation results can have a dramatic effect on subsequent simulation of the blood flow and the corresponding pressure landscape in the vessels. Since these results determine the decisions that the health providers take for a specific patient, Leo Grady encouraged the audience to not be satisfied with the evaluation scores accepted by the community but to aim at a clinical implementation of their methods and corresponding realistic accuracy targets. In a very interesting discussion, he described how a method proposed in one of the previous MICCAI conferences led to a highly relevant and successful business model that will likely impact a large number of patients.

The second invited talk was given by *Ron Kikinis* of Harvard Medical School, Cambridge, MA, USA. Ron Kikinis is widely known in the community for initiatives such as 3DSlicer. In his talk he highlighted the limitations inherent to the traditional academic research context that often leads to abandoned methods that never reach any clinical application. He called for a more focussed effort to connect algorithms developed in the medical image computing community to clinical users and their needs. Methods that are accepted by other researchers or clinicians have to have a crystal clear user interface, have to be fast and have to work in a different environment than the one they were developed for. He argued for *interactivity* of software tools as a central prerequisite for successful adoption of algorithms by health professionals. Often, efficient interaction is preferable to sub–optimal fully automatic analysis results. As a show case, he presented some of the features introduced in 3DSlicer based on the feedback by both developers and researchers and highlighted the importance of platforms that allow methods to be adaptable and improvable by other users, since they tend to have a higher impact in the community.

2.4   VISCERAL Section

The final session of the workshop focussed on VISCERAL. The goal of the session was to inform about the whole–body annotation benchmark, and kick–start a discussion among benchmark organizers and participants that is continuing after the workshop. After explaining the two benchmarks *Localization and segmentation* and *The surprise organ*, the audience was invited to discuss goals, analysis and possible extensions to cover as many relevant scenarios as possible, while staying a compact and concise challenge. This led to a discussion regarding the most important research challenges. The discussions addressed some of the obstacles of doing a multi–organ segmentation such as overcoming normal anatomical variability. Many participants showed an interest in a shared large dataset to compare their own approaches. Three approaches for organ segmentation and landmark detection were presented by HES–SO and Toshiba Medical Visualization Systems Europe who are registered participants of VISCERAL Benchmark 1.

In [14], the manually annotated volumes are registered to a new volume. This registration of several manually annotated volumes to a new volume allows to create probability maps for each of the organ in a flexible approach that does not use any a priori information. Such probability maps can then also be used for finding seed points for other segmentation algorithms, in this case the centroid of the highest probability map. In [21] a quite different approach is described by Jimenez et al. The presented work uses atlases for segmentation and can potentially be complementary to the text of Joyseeree et al. With atlases a priori information can be integrated into the segmentation process and thus relations between several organs are better modeled. Toshiba research presented and discussed their initial results of landmark detection, where they have internally a much larger data set than in the benchmark.

3   Conclusions

The third edition of the workshop on medical computer vision at MICCAI was a clear success. High quality papers and posters were presented and many discussions on scenarios and employed techniques emerged. It became clear that the domain still offers many research challenges. A particularly important topic is the handling and processing of large amounts of data which provides new challenges as well as new opportunities. The two presented challenges run through the EU–funded VISCERAL project support the research community in developing, validating and rating approaches by making a large data set of medical images publicly available and by providing an impartial evaluation framework. Such projects likely trigger changes for researchers in terms of validating approaches and developing novel algorithms that exploit the dense sampling of large data sets. While certain approaches work well for small–scale and specific problems, it might be entirely different approaches that best tackle issues emerging with large amounts of data. Clearly, this development is just at its beginning and we expect to see more exciting research arise from the community in the near future.

Acknowledgments. This work was supported by the EU in the FP7 through the VISCERAL (318068) and Khresmoi (257528) projects. The MCV best paper prizes were sponsored by Siemens Corporate Technology.

References

1. Abdelrehim, A., Farag, A., Shalaby, A., El-Melegy, M.: 2D-PCA shape models: application to 3D reconstruction of the human teeth from a single image. In: Menze, B., et al. (eds.): MCV 2013. LNCS, vol. 8331, pp. xx-yy. Springer, Heidelberg (2014)
2. Bauer, S., Tessier, J., Kreieter, O., Nolte, L.P., Reyes, M.: Integrated spatio-temporal segmentation of longitudinal brain tumor imaging studies. In: Menze, B., et al. (eds.): MCV 2013. LNCS, vol. 8331, pp. xx-yy. Springer, Heidelberg (2014)
3. Cabeen, R., Laidlaw, D.: White matter supervoxel segmentation by axial DP-means clustering. In: Menze, B., et al. (eds.): MCV 2013. LNCS, vol. 8331, pp. xx-yy. Springer, Heidelberg (2014)
4. Chou, C.R., Pizer, S.: Local regression learning via forest classification for 2D/3D deformable registration. In: Menze, B., et al. (eds.): MCV 2013. LNCS, vol. 8331, pp. xx-yy. Springer, Heidelberg (2014)
5. Chykeyuk, K., Noble, A.: Class-specific regression random forest for accurate extraction of standard planes from 3D echocardiography. In: Menze, B., et al. (eds.): MCV 2013. LNCS, vol. 8331, pp. xx-yy. Springer, Heidelberg (2014)

6. Corredor, G., Iregui, M., Arias, V., Romero, E.: Flexible architecture for streaming and visualization of large virtual microscopy images. In: Menze, B., et al. (eds.): MCV 2013. LNCS, vol. 8331, pp. xx-yy. Springer, Heidelberg (2014)
7. Domingos, J., Lima, E., Leeson, P., Noble, A.: Local phase-based fast ray features for automatic left ventricle apical view detection in 3D. In: Menze, B., et al. (eds.): MCV 2013. LNCS, vol. 8331, pp. xx-yy. Springer, Heidelberg (2014)
8. Gadermayr, M., Liedlgruber, M., Uhl, A., Vecsei, A.: Shape curvature histogram: a shape feature for celiac disease diagnosis. In: Menze, B., et al. (eds.): MCV 2013. LNCS, vol. 8331, pp. xx-yy. Springer, Heidelberg (2014)
9. Gadermayr, M., Uhl, A., Vecsei, A.: Feature extraction with intrincisc distortion correction in celiac disease imagery: no need for rasterization. In: Menze, B., et al. (eds.): MCV 2013. LNCS, vol. 8331, pp. xx-yy. Springer, Heidelberg (2014)
10. Galimzianova, A., Spiclin, T., Likar, B., Pernus, F.: Robust mixture-parameter estimation for unsupervised segmentation of brain MR images. In: Menze, B., et al. (eds.): MCV 2013. LNCS, vol. 8331, pp. xx-yy. Springer, Heidelberg (2014)
11. Ghesu, F., Wels, M., Jerebko, A., Suhling, M., Hornegger, J., Kelm, M.: Pectoral muscle detection in digital breast tomosyntheris and mammography. In: Menze, B., et al. (eds.): MCV 2013. LNCS, vol. 8331, pp. xx-yy. Springer, Heidelberg (2014)
12. Hafner, M., Uhl, A., Wimmer, G.: A novel shape feature descriptor for the classificatgion of polyps in HD coloscopy. In: Menze, B., et al. (eds.): MCV 2013. LNCS, vol. 8331, pp. xx-yy. Springer, Heidelberg (2014)
13. García Seco de Herrera, A., Foncubierta-Rodríguez, A., Schiavi, E., Müller, H.: 2D-based 3D volume retrieval using singular value docomposition of detected regions. In: Menze, B., et al. (eds.): MCV 2013. LNCS, vol. 8331, pp. xx-yy. Springer, Heidelberg (2014)
14. Joyseeree, R., Jiménez del Toro, O.A., Müller, H.: Using probability maps for multi-organ automatic segmentation. In: Menze, B., et al. (eds.): MCV 2013. LNCS, vol. 8331, pp. xx-yy. Springer, Heidelberg (2014)
15. Langs, G., Müller, H., Menze, B.H., Hanbury, A.: Visceral: Towards large data in medical imaging – challenges and directions. In: Menze, B., et al. (eds.): MCV 2013. LNCS, vol. 8331, pp. xx-yy. Springer, Heidelberg (2014)
16. Lu, L., Davarakota, P., Vikal, S., Wu, D., Zheng, Y., Wolf, M.: Computer aided diagnosis using multilevel image features on large-scale evaluation. In: MICCAI workshop on Medical Computer Vision. Lecture Notes in Computer Science, Springer (2013).
17. Menze, B.H., Langs, G., Lu, L., Montillo, A., Tu, Z., Criminisi, A. (eds.): MCV 2012. LNCS, vol. 7766. Springer, Heidelberg (2013)
18. Menze, B., Langs, G., Tu, Z., Criminisi, A. (eds.): MICCAI 2010. LNCS, vol. 6533. Springer, Heidelberg (2011)
19. Onofrey, J., Staib, L., Papademetris, X.: Semi-supervised learning of nonrigid deformations for image registration. In: Menze, B., et al. (eds.): MCV 2013. LNCS, vol. 8331, pp. xx-yy. Springer, Heidelberg (2014)
20. Song, Q., Montillo, A., Bhagalia, R., Srikrishnan: Organ localization using joint AP/LAT view landmark consensus detection and hierarchical active appearance models. In: Menze, B., et al. (eds.): MCV 2013. LNCS, vol. 8331, pp. xx-yy. Springer, Heidelberg (2014)
21. Jiménez del Toro, O.A., Müller, H.: Multi-structure atlasbased segmentation using anatomical regions of interest. In: Menze, B., et al. (eds.): MCV 2013. LNCS, vol. 8331, pp. xx-yy. Springer, Heidelberg (2014)

22. Wang, Q., Wu, D., Lu, L., Meizhu, L., Boyery, K., Zhou, K.: Semantic context forests for learning-based knee cartilage segmenrarion in 3D MR image. In: Menze, B., et al. (eds.): MCV 2013. LNCS, vol. 8331, pp. xx-yy. Springer, Heidelberg (2014)
23. Yan, Z., Zhang, S., Liu, Z., Metaxas, D., Montillo, A., AIBL: Accurate whole-brain segmentation for Alzheimer's disease combining an adaptive statistical atlas and multi-atlas. In: Menze, B., et al. (eds.): MCV 2013. LNCS, vol. 8331, pp. xx-yy. Springer, Heidelberg (2014)
24. Zheng, M., Carr, J., Ge, Y.: Automatic aorta detection in 3D cardiac CT images using bayesian tracking method. In: Menze, B., et al. (eds.): MCV 2013. LNCS, vol. 8331, pp. xx-yy. Springer, Heidelberg (2014)

Registration and Visualization

Semi-supervised Learning of Nonrigid Deformations for Image Registration

John A. Onofrey[1]($\boxtimes$), Lawrence H. Staib[1,2,3], and Xenophon Papademetris[1,3]

[1] Department of Biomedical Engineering, Yale University,
New Haven, CT 06520, USA
[2] Department of Electrical Engineering, Yale University, New Haven, CT 06520, USA
[3] Department of Diagnostic Radiology, Yale University, New Haven, CT 06520, USA
{john.onofrey,lawrence.staib,xenophon.papademetris}@yale.edu

Abstract. The existence of large medical image databases have made large amounts of neuroimaging data accessible and freely available to the research community. In this paper, we harness both the vast quantity of unlabeled anatomical MR brain scans from the 1000 Functional Connectomes Project (FCP1000) database and the smaller, but richly-annotated brain images from the LONI Probabilistic Brain Atlas (LPBA40) database to learn a statistical deformation model (SDM) of the nonrigid transformations in a semi-supervised learning (SSL) framework. We make use of 39 LPBA40 labeled MR datasets to create a set of supervised registrations and augment these results with a set of unsupervised registrations using 1247 unlabeled MRIs from the FCP1000. We show through leave-one-out cross validation that SSL of a nonrigid SDM results in a registration algorithm with significantly improved accuracy compared to standard, intensity-based registration, and does so with a 99 % reduction in transformation dimensionality.

Keywords: Image registration · Nonrigid · Semi-supervised learning · Statistical deformation model · Principal component analysis

1 Introduction

Nonrigid spatial normalization of different subjects to a common reference space has utility in a variety of medical imaging applications, for instance in population studies of functional brain imaging [5] and in atlas-based brain segmentation [1]. However, nonrigid image registration of different subjects is a challenging task made difficult, in part, by highly variable anatomical structure. Accurate anatomical alignment requires nonrigid transformations with a large number of degrees of freedom (DoFs). Inter-subject image registration with such high-dimensionality is an ill-posed optimization problem.

Statistical deformations models (SDMs) have the potential to reduce the dimensionality of the nonrigid transformations by learning the subspace or manifold in which these transformations exist. SDMs attempt to analyze anatomical

B. Menze et al. (Eds.): MCV 2013, LNCS 8331, pp. 13–23, 2014.
DOI: 10.1007/978-3-319-05530-5_2, © Springer International Publishing Switzerland 2014

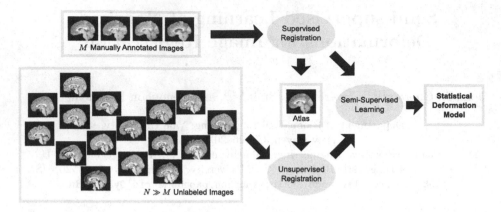

Fig. 1. Our semi-supervised learning approach makes use of both a small number of gold-standard, manually-annotated image samples and a large number of unlabeled image samples. We use the labeled VOIs in the M annotated images to perform a type of supervised nonrigid registration, from which we create a reference atlas composed of average anatomy and majority-vote label images. We then nonrigidly register the N unlabeled images to the atlas in an unsupervised manner using standard, intensity-only registration. Finally, we perform a principal component analysis of the supervised and unsupervised transformations to learn a statistical deformation model.

variation by modeling the nonrigid image deformations from a set of training images. Rueckert *et al.* [10] proposed principal component analysis (PCA) of nonrigid deformations to create a low-dimensional, linear orthonormal basis of high-dimensional registrations. Other authors have made use of PCA-based SDMs in this manner for low-dimensional image registration [7] and as a registration regularization prior [15]. However, if the SDM is not trained using accurate registrations, the utility of the model is questionable. Onofrey *et al.* [8] demonstrate improved PCA SDM performance by training with a set of richly-annotated images. Regardless of training the SDM with labeled or unlabeled data, previous PCA-based SDMs offer relatively underwhelming registration performance due to PCA's inability to model the high-dimensional transformation's variance with orders of magnitude fewer number of training samples.

Thankfully, large medical image databases containing vast amounts of neuroimaging data, such as the 1000 Functional Connectomes Project International Neuroimaging Data-Sharing Initiative [2] (FCP1000), offer an accessible and freely available source of SDM training samples. In contrast, smaller databases like the UCLA Laboratory of Neuroimaging (LONI) Probabilistic Brain Atlas (LPBA40) [12] contain relatively few images, but incorporate richly-annotated information, such as gold-standard manually-segmented volumes of interest (VOIs). Datasets containing such rich information are labor intensive and expensive to create. In this paper, we leverage both the vast quantity of unlabeled anatomical MR brain scans from the FCP1000 dataset and the small, but labeled brain images from the LPBA40 dataset to learn a SDM of nonrigid registration in a semi-supervised learning (SSL) framework. The concepts of using both labeled and unlabeled training data for SSL are widely applicable for classification problems [3], but its use for image registration is novel, to the best of our knowledge. As illustrated in Fig. 1, we make use of 39 of the LPBA40's labeled MR datasets to create a set of supervised registrations. We augment this supervised sample set with a second set of unsupervised registrations using 1247 unlabeled MRIs from the FCP1000. To the best of our knowledge, no prior work has made use 1286 MRIs to learn a SDM for image registration. We show through leave-one-out cross validation that semi-supervised learning (SSL) our nonrigid statistical deformation model (SDM) results in a nonrigid registration algorithm with significantly improved accuracy compared to standard, intensity-based registration, and does so with a 99 % reduction in transformation dimensionality.

2   Methods

Our proposed SSL nonrigid registration framework requires both supervised and unsupervised training registration samples. For both types of registrations, we use a free-form deformation (FFD) transformation model [11]. The FFD B-spline control point displacements parameterize a dense nonrigid deformation field $T(\mathbf{x}) \in \mathbb{R}^3$ at all voxels $\mathbf{x} \in \Omega \subset \mathbb{R}^3$, where Ω is the reference image volume in three dimensions. We rewrite this transformation as a column vector of P concatenated FFD control point displacements, $\mathbf{d} \in \mathbb{R}^{3P}$.

We denote the set of nonrigid transformations computed using a *supervised* registration procedure $D_s = \{\mathbf{d}_m | m = 1, \ldots, M\}$ and the set of nonrigid transformations estimated using an *unsupervised* registration approach $D_u = \{\mathbf{d}_{M+n} | n = 1, \ldots, N\}$. Sections 2.1 and 2.2 describe our supervised and unsupervised registration methodologies, respectively. We registered all $M+N$ sample images to a common reference space (described in Sect. 2.1) with $181 \times 217 \times 181$ volume with $1\,\mathrm{mm}^3$ resolution. For an FFD with 5 mm control point spacing, this volume required $P = 60,236$ control points, thus each deformation had 180,708 DoFs in 3D. Together, the sets D_s and D_u comprise our SDM's SSL training set. Section 2.3 describes our SDM and how we subsequently used that SDM to nonrigidly register images not included in the training set.

2.1   Supervised Nonrigid Registration

To create our set of supervised nonrigid registrations D_s, we make use of a database containing gold-standard, manually-segmented VOIs to constrain our deformations with respect to these VOIs [8]. The LPBA40 database [12] contains 40 anatomical, skull-stripped brain MR images I_i, $i = 1, \ldots, 40$, with 56 annotated VOIs. In order to calculate our nonrigid registrations using a common reference domain, we first register all 40 images to the MNI Colin 27 brain. We then select subject 1 to be used as an initial reference template image I_1 for nonrigid registration of the remaining subjects. Using an integrated intensity and point-feature nonrigid registration algorithm [9], we nonrigidly register the remaining $M = 39$ subjects to our reference. This algorithm uses a FFD transformation model with 5 mm control point spacing and minimizes the sum of squared differences (SSD) similarity measure while penalizing misalignment of the VOI surface points according to the robust point matching algorithm [4]. The labeled image data allows for accurate normalization of anatomical image intensities, which motivates using SSD for these registrations. We denote these transformations $T_{i \rightsquigarrow 1}, i = 2, \ldots, 40$ ($i \rightsquigarrow j$ denotes nonrigid registration from space i to j). Our choice of reference image biases the registrations to that subject's particular anatomy. To correct for this, we compute the mean transformation $\bar{T} = \frac{1}{M} \sum_{i=2}^{40} T_{i \rightsquigarrow 1}$ and apply the inverse transformation $\bar{T}^{-1}$ to subject 1 to create a deformation bias-corrected (DBC) image $I_{\mathrm{DBC}} = \bar{T}^{-1} \circ I_1$, where $\circ$ is the transformation operator. We then re-register the M subjects to I_{DBC} using the same integrated nonrigid registration as before, and denote these transformations $T_{i \rightsquigarrow \mathrm{DBC}}$. As this set of transformations leverages annotated VOIs and we constrain our registration procedure to align these VOIs, the FFD control point displacements of these transformations constitute our set of supervised registrations $D_s = \{\mathbf{d}_m | m = 1, \ldots, M\}$.

In addition to creating D_s, we also create an atlas composed of an anatomical image $I_{\mathrm{Atlas}} = \frac{1}{M-1} \sum_{i=2}^{40} T_{i \rightsquigarrow \mathrm{DBC}} \circ I_i$ and a corresponding VOI label image found using a majority-vote of the 39 transformed subject VOIs. I_{Atlas} is a representative template image for the set of nonrigid FFD transformations with 5 mm control point spacing. We thus use I_{Atlas} as the reference image for our unsupervised registrations described in the following section.

2.2 Unsupervised Nonrigid Registration

We require a large number of unsupervised samples to supplement our small set of supervised registrations. From the FCP1000 database [2], we culled $N = 1247$ unlabeled, anatomical brain MR images of healthy, normal subjects. First, we register all images to our common reference space, I_{Atlas}, using an affine transformation $T_{n \rightarrow \mathrm{Atlas}}, n = 1, \ldots, N$ ($i \rightarrow j$ denotes rigid registration from space i to j) by maximizing the normalized mutual information (NMI) similarity metric [13]. Following affine registration, we then estimate the nonrigid deformation of all N brains to I_{Atlas}.

Using the same FFD nonrigid transformation model with 5 mm control point spacing as in Sect. 2.1, we nonrigidly register each subject by maximizing NMI. However, unlike the skull-stripped LPBA40 images in Sect. 2.1, these images have no manual correction, and thus artifacts, e.g. the optic nerve, remain in some images (as can be seen in Fig. 1). Such artifacts present challenges for intensity-based registration methods. Rather than manually correcting these poor segmentations, we perform weighted nonrigid registration [14] that preferentially weights the brain region during the calculation of NMI. For this, we create a brain weight mask image by first dilating I_{Atlas}'s brain mask and then smoothing with a Gaussian kernel. The resulting transformations $T_{n \rightsquigarrow \mathrm{Atlas}}$ and their respective FFD control point displacements comprise our set of unsupervised registrations $D_u = \{\mathbf{d}_{M+n} | n = 1, \ldots, N\}$.

2.3   Semi-supervised Statistical Deformation Model Registration

Using both the supervised and unsupervised registration sets, D_s and D_u, respectively, we create a statistical deformation model (SDM) of nonrigid FFD transformation [10]. A principal component analysis of the deformations $\mathbf{d}_i, i = 1, \ldots, M + N$ gives a linear approximation of the deformation distribution

$$\mathbf{d} = \bar{\mathbf{d}} + \Phi \mathbf{w} \tag{1}$$

where $\bar{\mathbf{d}} = \frac{1}{M+N} \sum_{i=1}^{M+N} \mathbf{d}_i$ is the mean deformation of the $M + N$ training registrations, $\Phi = (\phi_1 | \ldots | \phi_K) \in \mathbb{R}^{3P \times K}$ is the matrix of orthogonal eigenvectors, and $\mathbf{w} \in \mathbb{R}^K$ is a vector of model coefficients. The number of training samples determines the number of eigenvectors such that $K = \min\{M + N, 3P\}$. The k-th eigenvalue λ_k estimates the sample variance along the eigenvector ϕ_k, and we sort them in decreasing order $\lambda_1 \geq \lambda_2 \geq \ldots \geq \lambda_K$. A SDM using K_v parameters accounts for $0 \leq v \leq 100\,\%$ of the model's cumulative variance

$$\sum_{k=1}^{K_v} \lambda_k \leq v \sum_{k=1}^{K} \lambda_k.$$

Thus, using the first K_v coefficients of $\mathbf{w}$ in Eq. 1 provides a low-dimensional parameterization (K_v DoFs) of a high-dimensional FFD $\mathbf{d}$, which we denote $T_{\mathrm{SDM}_v}(\mathbf{x}; \mathbf{w})$ for all points $\mathbf{x}$ in the reference image domain Ω.

To nonrigidly register a new image I to our reference image I_{Atlas}, we use the SDM from Eq. 1 to optimize the cost function

$$\hat{T}_{\mathrm{SDM}_v} = \arg \max_{\mathbf{w}} J(I_{\mathrm{Atlas}}, T_{\mathrm{SDM}_v}(\cdot; \mathbf{w}) \circ I). \tag{2}$$

Here, J is the NMI similarity metric evaluated throughout the image volume. We solve Eq. 2 using conjugate gradient optimization with a hierarchical multi-resolution image pyramid.

3   Results and Discussion

We tested our SSL SDM by performing a series of *leave-one-out* tests. For each supervised registration $\mathbf{d}_i \in D_s$, we recomputed the SDM in Sect. 2.3 by leaving the i-th deformation out of Eq. 1. We did not recompute I_{Atlas} as in Sect. 2.1 for each leave-one-out test because the single subject's exclusion had negligible effect on the mean intensity image. Section 3.1 presents results showing the SDM's ability to reconstruct each of the $i = 1, \ldots, 39$ deformations. Section 3.2 then shows how well the SDM registered $\mathbf{d}_i$'s corresponding anatomical image I_i in the LPBA40 dataset to I_{Atlas} using Eq. 2. For comparison, we created another SDM using standard, unsupervised-only registration training samples. We trained this unsupervised SDM with $N + M$ training samples by replacing the LPBA40 supervised registrations in D_s with unsupervised registrations of the same images using our methodology from Sect. 2.2. We also compared our results to standard, intensity-only FFD registration using 5 mm control point spacing, which we denote FFD_5.

To evaluate registration accuracy in both sections, we calculated the mean Dice overlap (MDO) of the $V = 56$ VOIs with respect to the atlas labels

$$\mathrm{MDO}_i = \frac{1}{V} \sum_{v \in V} \frac{2|(I_i)_v \cap (I_{\mathrm{Atlas}})_v|}{|(I_i)_v| + |(I_{\mathrm{Atlas}})_v|}$$

where $(A)_v$ denotes the v-th VOI from image A. We found MDO to be a suitable summary statistic to quantify registration performance rather than analyze each individual VOI Dice overlap separately. Furthermore, since our supervised registration framework constrained VOI boundaries to align and a certain amount of registration uncertainty remains at locations away from those boundaries, our use of Dice overlap more appropriately measures accurate alignment of VOI boundaries than a residual sum of square transformation error.

We implemented our code on the GPU using the CUDA parallel programming platform as part of BioImage Suite [6]. The eigensystem in Eq. 1 may be precomputed ahead of the registration, and can then be loaded into the algorithm to avoid unnecessarily repetitive PCA computation. We compared the computation time of our approach to standard FFD_5.

3.1 SSL SDM Reconstructions

For each leave-one-out test, we tested the SDM's ability to reconstruct the i-th subject's deformation $\mathbf{d}_i$ by rewriting Eq. 1 and solving

$$\hat{\mathbf{d}}_i = \bar{\mathbf{d}}_i + \boldsymbol{\Phi}_i \boldsymbol{\Phi}_i^T (\mathbf{d}_i - \bar{\mathbf{d}}_i)$$

where $\hat{\mathbf{d}}_i$ is a least-squares approximation to $\mathbf{d}_i$, and we calculated $\bar{\mathbf{d}}_i$ and $\boldsymbol{\Phi}_i$ using $\mathbf{d}_j, \forall j \neq i$. We resliced image I_i using $\hat{\mathbf{d}}_i$ and computed the MDO_i. Figure 2 compares the reconstruction performance of the SSL SDM and the unsupervised SDM using different numbers of unsupervised registration training samples, $0 \leq N \leq 1247$. We selected the N samples sequentially, without randomization. Figure 2 also shows how the SSL SDMs performed using only supervised samples, i.e. $N = 0$.

As to be expected, reconstruction performance increased with the number of samples. However, the inclusion of only a small number of supervised registration samples, $M = 38$ in the case of leave-one-out testing, significantly increased the reconstructive capabilities of the SDM. This observed increase in SDM reconstruction performance is the result of the supervised training samples increasing the PCA model space's variance. Using standard FFD_5 registration as a reference for comparison (MDO $= 78.09 \pm 1.26$, shown in Table 1), the SSL SDM had approximately the same level of registration performance using $N = 400$ unsupervised samples, and significantly better performance using the full $N = 1247$ unsupervised samples. On the other hand, the unsupervised SDM required $N = 1285$ samples to achieve the equivalent performance as FFD_5.

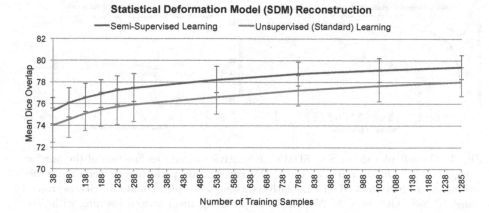

Fig. 2. Mean dice overlap values for leave-one-out transformation reconstructions as a function of the number of training samples. The inclusion of a few, 39, supervised registration samples significantly increased the SDM's reconstruction abilities. These results represent an upper bound for SDM registration performance. The plotted values are the mean with error bars of one standard deviation.

We also noted that the MDO curves in Fig. 2 appeared to be continuing to increase with inclusion of additional training samples. These reconstructions provided a theoretical upper bound for SDM registration performance, and Sect. 3.2 presents how well our proposed SDM effectively registered images in practice.

3.2   SSL SDM Registration

Having shown theoretical improvements, we now demonstrate that our approach also works in practice. For each of the 39 leave-one-out test cases, we compared registration using 4 methods: (i) SSL SDM with $M = 38, N = 1247$ training samples, (ii) unsupervised SDM with $M = 0, N = 1285$ training samples, (iii) supervised SDM with $M = 38, N = 0$ training samples, and (iv) standard, intensity FFD$_5$. For each of the SDM's, we registered I_i using the first K_v eigenvectors that contained the first $v = 25, 50, 75, 90, 95, 99, 100\%$ percentage of variance (for the supervised SDM, we replaced $v = 25$ with 33% to avoid using 0 eigenvectors) and computed MDO$_i$. For each percentage of variance v, SSL SDM required $K_v = 5, 19, 76, 228, 390, 800, 1285$ eigenvectors, respectively, as shown on the left of Fig. 3. Similarly, the unsupervised SDM required $K_v = 4, 19, 77, 236, 405, 817, 1285$ eigenvectors and the supervised SDM required $K_v = 1, 2, 11, 23, 29, 35, 38$ eigenvectors. The number of eigenvectors defined the dimensionality of the nonrigid deformation. Figure 3 plots the cumulative variance v of the SSL SDM as function of the number of eigenvectors used, K_v.

Figure 3 also shows MDO as function of v for each of the three SDM types. As seen in Sect. 3.1, SSL SDM significantly outperformed unsupervised SDM for all values of v ($p \leq 8.9 \times 10^{-8}$, two-tailed paired t-test). The supervised SDM performed worse than both SSL and unsupervised SDMs, with the exception

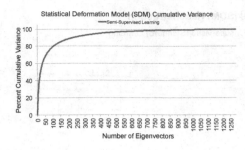
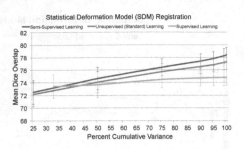

Fig. 3. The left plot shows SSL SDM's cumulative variance as function of the number of eigenvectors. On the right, we show SDM registration performance using mean dice overlap as a function of SDM cumulative variance. We plot results for SDMs trained using: (i) SSL with $M = 38, N = 1247$ samples, (ii) unsupervised learning with $N = 1285$ samples, and (iii) supervised learning with $M = 38$ samples.

Table 1. Leave-one-out registration results comparing our proposed SSL SDM registration method using 100 % of the variance, i.e. all PCA eigenvectors, with SDMs using supervised and unsupervised training samples alone, as well as standard, intensity FFD registration using 5 mm control point spacing. Reported values are mean±std MDO and minimum MDO for 39 subjects. Computational times were measured using an NVIDIA GeForce GTX 580 GPU.

Method	DoFs	MDO	Min MDO	Compute Time (m)
SSL SDM	1285	**78.35 ± 1.19**	**75.90**	36.62 ± 7.60
Unsupervised SDM	1285	77.28 ± 1.22	73.85	33.10 ± 5.74
Supervised SDM	38	74.77 ± 1.23	70.83	0.55 ± 0.07
Intensity FFD$_5$	180,708	78.09 ± 1.26	74.08	73.85 ± 1.39

of using $v = 0.33$, i.e. a single eigenvector. These results were to be expected given the small number of training samples, $M = 38$, and the large percentage of cumulative variance modeled by the first eigenvector. However, we observed that the SSL SDM was unable to fully achieve the theoretical reconstructive performance of the SDM. While our registration algorithm's performance closely followed that of the SSL reconstructions, our use of NMI as a similarity metric appeared to yield a non-convex cost function with local minima that prevented our algorithm from attaining the SDM's theoretical performance bound at a global minimum.

Table 1 highlights the results of our tests using $v = 100\%$ for each of the registration methods. In terms of MDO, our SSL SDM performed significantly better than FFD$_5$, unsupervised SDM, and supervised SDM using two-tailed, paired t-tests ($p \leq 0.02$). Most impressively, the SDM achieved more accurate registration than FFD$_5$ while reducing the dimensionality of the nonrigid deformation from 180,708 to 1285, a 99 % reduction in DoFs. This translated to a 50 % speedup in mean computation time. Also of note is SSL SDM's worst case performance, with minimum MDO 75.90, being higher than FFD$_5$'s minimum

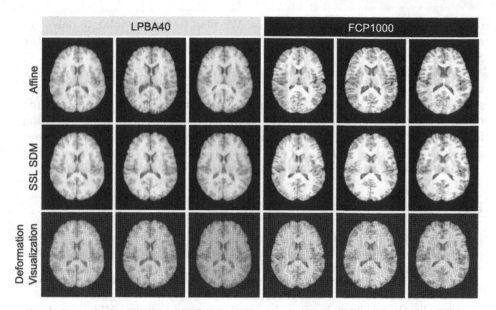

Fig. 4. Exemplar subjects and their respective registrations using our semi-supervised learning (SSL) SDM during leave-one-out tests. We show example images drawn from both the supervised (LPBA40) and unsupervised (FCP1000) training datasets. The first row shows the original images after affine registration to our atlas reference (not pictured). The second row shows the same images after SSL SDM registration using 1285 eigenvectors. The third row overlays a 5 mm isotropic grid to visualize the nonrigid deformation.

MDO 74.08. By constraining the registration transformation to be from the learned space of deformations, the SDM prevented the registration from becoming stuck in worse local minima. Figure 4 illustrates the SSL SDM registration results for some exemplar images drawn from both the supervised (LPBA40) and unsupervised (FCP1000) training data.

4   Conclusion

We demonstrate the utility of using an existing large-scale medical image database to augment the learning of nonrigid SDMs. By training a SDM in a semi-supervised manner using both a small set of accurate, supervised registrations and a large set of registrations of unknown quality, we show significantly improved registration performance with a 99 % reduction in registration DoFs. The constraints afforded by the learned SDM not only serve to better register images but also to avoid poor registration that could otherwise occur with unconstrained and unsupervised registration algorithms. While our registration algorithm in Eq. 2 does not bias the deformations towards the mean deformation, it may be of interest to implement the algorithm in a Bayesian framework and compare registration performance and robustness. We plan to further validate our algorithm using other databases that contain annotated brain images and to test the SDM's generalizability.

Our future work aims to explore methods for nonlinear dimensionality reduction, and compare these results to that of linear PCA. However, the results presented in this paper show that, while simple, PCA is indeed effective at modeling the high-dimensional space of nonrigid brain deformations, and that the limiting factor for a PCA-based SDM is the number of training samples used. Both our theoretical and actual SSL SDM registration results suggest that the space of nonrigid deformations between subjects is of surprisingly low dimensionality.

References

1. Aljabar, P., Heckemann, R., Hammers, A., Hajnal, J., Rueckert, D.: Multi-atlas based segmentation of brain images: atlas selection and its effect on accuracy. NeuroImage **46**(3), 726–738 (2009)
2. Biswal, B.B., et al.: Toward discovery science of human brain function. Proc. Nat. Acad. Sci. **107**(10), 4734–4739 (2010)
3. Chapelle, O., Schölkopf, B., Zien, A.: Semi-supervised Learning. MIT Press, Cambridge (2006)
4. Chui, H., Rangarajan, A.: A new point matching algorithm for non-rigid registration. Comput. Vis. Image Underst. **89**(2–3), 114–141 (2003)
5. Gholipour, A., Kehtarnavaz, N., Briggs, R., Devous, M., Gopinath, K.: Brain functional localization: a survey of image registration techniques. IEEE Trans. Med. Imaging **26**(4), 427–451 (2007)
6. Joshi, A., Scheinost, D., Okuda, H., Belhachemi, D., Murphy, I., Staib, L., Papademetris, X.: Unified framework for development, deployment and robust testing of neuroimaging algorithms. Neuroinformatics **9**, 69–84 (2011)
7. Kim, M.J., Kim, M.H., Shen, D.: Learning-based deformation estimation for fast non-rigid registration. In: IEEE Computer Society Conference on Computer Vision and Pattern Recognition Workshops, 2008, CVPRW '08, pp. 1–6 (June 2008)
8. Onofrey, J., Staib, L., Papademetris, X.: Fast nonrigid registration using statistical deformation models learned from richly annotated data. In: 2013 IEEE International Symposium on Biomedical Imaging: From Nano to Macro, pp. 576–579 (April 2013)
9. Papademetris, X., Jackowski, A.P., Schultz, R.T., Staib, L.H., Duncan, J.S.: Integrated intensity and point-feature nonrigid registration. In: Barillot, C., Haynor, D.R., Hellier, P. (eds.) MICCAI 2004. LNCS, vol. 3216, pp. 763–770. Springer, Heidelberg (2004)
10. Rueckert, D., Frangi, A., Schnabel, J.: Automatic construction of 3-D statistical deformation models of the brain using nonrigid registration. IEEE Trans. Med. Imaging **22**(8), 1014–1025 (2003)
11. Rueckert, D., Sonoda, L., Hayes, C., Hill, D., Leach, M., Hawkes, D.: Nonrigid registration using free-form deformations: application to breast MR images. IEEE Trans. Med. Imaging **18**(8), 712–721 (1999)
12. Shattuck, D., et al.: Construction of a 3D probabilistic atlas of human cortical structures. NeuroImage **39**(3), 1064–1080 (2008)
13. Studholme, C., Hill, D., Hawkes, D.: An overlap invariant entropy measure of 3D medical image alignment. Pattern Recogn. **32**(1), 71–86 (1999)

14. Suh, J., Scheinost, D., Qian, X., Sinusas, A.J., Breuer, C., Papademetris, X.: Serial nonrigid vascular registration using weighted normalized mutual information. In: 2010 IEEE International Symposium on Biomedical Imaging: From Nano to Macro, pp. 25–28 (2010)
15. Xue, Z., Shen, D., Davatzikos, C.: Statistical representation of high-dimensional deformation fields with application to statistically constrained 3D warping. Med. Image Anal. **10**(5), 740–751 (2006)

Local Regression Learning via Forest Classification for 2D/3D Deformable Registration

Chen-Rui Chou[✉] and Stephen Pizer

Department of Computer Science, University of North Carolina at Chapel Hill,
Chapel Hill, USA
cchou@cs.unc.edu

Abstract. Recent 2D/3D deformable registration methods have achieved real-time computation of 3D lung deformations by learning global regressions that map projection intensities to deformation parameters globally in a shape space. If the mapping matrices are specialized to a specific local region of the shape space, the linear mappings will perform better than mappings trained to work on the global shape space. The major contribution of this paper is presenting a novel method that supports *shape-space-localized* learning for 2D/3D deformable registration and uses regression learning as an example. The method comprises two stages: training and application. In the training stage, it recursively finds normalized graph cuts that best separate the training samples given the number of desired training partitions. Second, in each training partition the projection mapping matrices are learned by linear regressions locally. Third, the method trains a decision forest for deciding into which training partition a target projection image should be classified, on the basis of projection image intensity and gradient values in various image regions. In the application stage, the decision forest classifies a target projection image into a training partition and then the learned linear regressions for that training partition are applied to the target projection image intensities to yield the desired deformation. This local regression learning method is validated on both synthetic and real lung datasets. The results indicate that the forest classification followed by local regressions yields more accurate and yet still real-time 2D/3D deformable registration than global regressions.

1 Introduction

Regression learning has been a simple but efficacious way to understand the relationship between medical images and medical facts. In medical image registration, regression learning provides a way to understand patients' deformations from their medical images such that the calculated deformation can be constrained to a previously learned space instead of an arbitrary one. However, means to optimize the regression learning for registration efficiency and accuracy have not been well-addressed. This paper investigates a learning variation

B. Menze et al. (Eds.): MCV 2013, LNCS 8331, pp. 24–33, 2014.
DOI: 10.1007/978-3-319-05530-5_3, © Springer International Publishing Switzerland 2014

to the registration efficiency and accuracy for one of the medical applications - lung Image-Guided Radiation Therapy (IGRT).

The goal of lung IGRT is to place the radiation beam on the ever-changing tumor centroid under the patient's respiratory motion while avoiding organs at risks (OAR). One way to accomplish this goal is by 2D/3D image registration. 2D/3D image registration computes the patient's 3D treatment-time deformation vector fields (DVFs) by registering the patient's treatment-time imaging x-ray projection image to the patient's planning-time 3D CT image. If the DVFs can be computed accurately and in real time, the computed DVFs not only can guide physicians to make medical decision within treatment fractions, the DVFs at the radiation deliveries can also be used for the inter-fraction dose accumulation study for adaptive therapy.

Recent learning-based 2D/3D registration approaches [1,2] have shown promise in real-time registration. In order to obtain acceptable registration accuracy, both approaches constrain the registration computation to a patient-specific deformation shape space analyzed from the patient's treatment-planning Respiratory-Correlated CTs (RCCTs). Specifically, [1] learned global linear regressions that map projection intensities to their associated deformation parameters based on a sampling from the whole deformation space. At treatment time the learned patient-specific regressions are iteratively applied to refine the estimation of the patient's deformation parameters. Reference [2] presented an even faster regression learning method that does not need to iterate for refinement. It estimates the patient's deformation parameters by learning optimal global projection distance metrics for deformation parameter interpolation via nonlinear kernel regressions.

However, due to the variable projection-to-deformation relationships in various regions of the deformation space, a global regression or a global distance metric learned from the whole deformation space is a rough approximation of the underlying relationship. As a result, the registration accuracy is limited by the global learning methods.

This paper presents a novel local learning method that partitions the shape space, learns a projection-to-deformation relationship for each partition and at application time applies the learned local relationship of a classified partition to yield better approximation. The method improves the regression learning method described in [1] as an example. The results show that the method's local regression learning yields a more accurate and yet still real-time 2D/3D deformable registration.

Specifically, the method generates large-scale training samples and finds normalized graph cuts [3] that best separate the training samples into a given number of training partitions. In each training partition the method learns linear regression matrices that map the training projection intensities to the training deformation parameters. At treatment time, the method decides which training partition the target deformation resides in by a trained decision forest ([4], an approach that has shown success in many medical applications) based on projection image intensities and gradients of various image regions in the target projection image. The linear regressions learned for the forest-decided partition are applied to the target projection intensities to yield the desired deformation.

2 Method

The purpose of the local regression learning is to obtain a better regression fitting to the training set. Due to the nonlinear relationships between the deformation parameters and the projection intensities, fitting a globally linear regression to approximate this nonlinear relationship is mathematically inappropriate. This section presents a locally-linear regression learning method that can approximate this nonlinear relationship. It comprises two stages: training and treatment application. There are five steps in the training stage. First, the patient's prior deformation space is parameterized by an LDDMM (Large Deformation Diffeomorphic Metric Mapping) framework from the patient's treatment-planning RCCTs. Second, the method samples training deformation parameters and simulates corresponding x-ray projection images, or DRRs (Digitally-Reconstructed Radiographs), from CT volumes warped by the sampled training deformations. Third, the method partitions the training projection images recursively by normalized graph cuts using Euclidean distances of the deformation parameters. Fourth, the method fits a linear regression between the deformation parameters and the covarying projection intensities for each training partition. Finally, in order to classify an unseen projection image into a nearest training partition in the treatment application stage, in the training stage the method trains a set of decision trees, or a decision forest, for deciding the local training partition based on the projection image intensities and gradients of various image regions. In the treatment application stage, given a target projection image the method estimates the deformation parameters of the patient by first classifying the target projection image into a training partition and then using the learned linear regression of that partition to yield the estimation.

2.1 Training Stage

Deformation Space Formulation. The method uses the same deformation space formulation as described in [1,2]. The method constrains the patient's deformation to a space spanned from the deformation observed in the patient's treatment-planning RCCTs. The RCCTs consist of 10 phase images. From those 10 phase images, a respiratory Fréchet mean, as well as the diffeomorphic deformations ϕ_τ from the mean to each image J_τ with phase τ, are computed by an LDDMM framework. With the diffeomorphic deformation set $\{\phi_\tau\}_{\tau=1,2,\cdots,10}$ calculated, the method finds a mean deformation $\overline{\phi}$ and a set of linear deformation eigenmodes ϕ_{pc}^i by PCA analysis. The weights λ_τ^i on each deformation eigenmode i yield a deformation ϕ_τ in terms of these deformation eigenmodes: $\phi_\tau = \overline{\phi} + \sum_{i=1}^{10} \lambda_\tau^i \cdot \phi_{pc}^i$. For most of the target problems the first three eigenmodes capture more than 95 % of the total variations observed among the RCCTs. The first three eigenmode weights then form an 3-dimensional parametrization $\mathbf{c}$ of the patient's deformation space: $\mathbf{c} = (c^1, c^2, c^3) = (\lambda^1, \lambda^2, \lambda^3)$.

Training Space Sampling. The method uniformly samples S weights on each deformation eigenmode within ± 3 standard deviations of the eigenmode weights observed in the planning RCCTs. For 3-dimensional parametrization of the deformation space, a total $N = S^3$ sampled deformation parameters $\{\mathbf{c}_\kappa\}_{\kappa=1,2,...,N}$ are used to warp the Fréchet mean image, and the training projection images $\{\mathbf{P}_\kappa\}_{\kappa=1,2,...,N}$ are simulated from those warped mean images. Particularly, in order to make the intensity comparable between the training projections and treatment-time target projections, the method normalizes both training and target projections with a local Gaussian normalization method described in [1].

Training Space Partitioning. To partition the training projections, the method uses a hierarchical separation approach that is similar to the normalized graphs cut method [3]. The goal of the training space partitioning is to separate the training space such that the Euclidean distance of the deformation parameters in each partition is minimized. Different than the traditional graph cut approach that generates an "affinity" matrix, the method generates an $N \times N$ "dissimilarity" matrix $\mathcal{D}$ where the entries $\mathcal{D}_{i,j} = \|\mathbf{c}_i - \mathbf{c}_j\|_2$ are the distances of the deformation eigenmode weights between training samples i and j. N is the number of training samples. Having the dissimilarity matrix computed, the method computes the first k smallest eigenvalues and their eigenvectors $V_1, V_2, .., V_k$ of the dissimilarity matrix $\mathcal{D}$ if 2^k partitions are needed. The eigenvector with the smallest eigenvalue, V_1, is an approximation to the NP-hard normalized graph cut problem [3]: training samples close to each other will have similar values in the eigenvector (have close dissimilarity maps). Therefore, the method sorts the training samples by their values in V_1 and partitions the training samples into two by the median value. The final partitioning can be computed by recursively separating the training set using the eigenvectors with the next smallest eigenvalues.

Local Regression Learning. The method approximates the nonlinear relationship between the projection intensities and the deformation parameters by fitting a linear regression $\mathbf{W}_{\mathcal{L}}^i$ that linearly maps the projection intensities to the ith deformation parameter $c_{\kappa \in \mathcal{L}}^i$ for each training sample κ in each local training partition $\mathcal{L}$ (local deformation neighborhood): $c_{\kappa \in \mathcal{L}}^i \approx \mathbf{P}_{\kappa \in \mathcal{L}} \cdot \mathbf{W}_{\mathcal{L}}^i$ where $\mathbf{W}_{\mathcal{L}}^i = (\mathbf{P}_{\kappa \in \mathcal{L}}^\mathsf{T} \cdot \mathbf{P}_{\kappa \in \mathcal{L}})^{-1} \cdot \mathbf{P}_{\kappa \in \mathcal{L}}^\mathsf{T} \cdot c_{\kappa \in \mathcal{L}}^i$.

Decision Forest Training. In order to efficiently classify an unseen target projection into a training partition in the application stage, the method constructs a decision forest $\mathcal{F}$ in the training stage. The decision forest $\mathcal{F}$ consists of M binary trees $\mathcal{T}_1, \mathcal{T}_2, .., \mathcal{T}_M$ with depth d. In this paper $M = 100$ and $d = 5$ are used. In each tree, a tree traversal of the target projection selects the nearest training projection images. With the 100 tree traversals the method classifies the target projection image into the same partition as its most frequently selected nearest training projection image's. The tree traversal is guided by a sequence of binary decisions made at tree nodes based on the "visual features" of the target projection image. The visual features used in this paper are 6 features: mean intensity, mean intensity difference, mean intensity gradients along two projection axes, and mean intensity gradient differences along two projection axes of $1,000$ random box pairs (random positions and sizes).

The method constructs such a decision forest through a supervised learning on the training set: In each tree the binary decisions made at tree nodes are to select visual features and their thresholds to partition the training projection images such that training projection images with close deformation parameter values will traverse to the same leaf node. Specifically, for each binary tree T_δ the method randomly selects 400 candidate visual features V_δ out of the total $1,000 \times 6 = 6,000$ visual features V. At each tree node N in the tree T_δ the method selects the qth visual feature V_N^q among the 150 candidate visual features V_N randomly sampled from V_δ ($V_N^q \in V_N \subset V_\delta \subset V$) and the threshold ξ for the selected visual feature V_N^q such that after the binary partition by the threshold, the total variance of the deformation parameters is minimized or equivalently, the information gain is maximized: for training samples κ in tree node N,

$$\underset{q,\xi}{\textbf{argmax}}\ \textbf{Var}\{c_{\kappa\in N}\} - \textbf{Var}\{c_{\kappa\in N}|V_N^q(\mathbf{P}_\kappa) \geqslant \xi\} - \textbf{Var}\{c_{\kappa\in N}|V_N^q(\mathbf{P}_\kappa) < \xi\} \quad (1)$$

With optimizations (1) at all tree nodes in all trees, training projection images traverse to the same leaf nodes in a tree have the same visual feature responses to the binary decisions and similar deformation parameter values. The random selection of the candidate features for each tree and for each node provides an efficient and robust discriminative learning from the high dimensional feature space [5]. The method records the leaf node indices where the training projection images visited in each tree for classification in the treatment application stage.

2.2   Treatment Application Stage

In the treatment application stage, an unseen target projection image is preprocessed to remove the additional photon scattering with a local Gaussian normalization method described in [1]. The method then classifies the target projection image into a local training partition by the trained regression forest. Finally, the target deformation parameters are estimated by the local linear regressions learned from that local partition. With the efficient forest classification and the fast parameter estimation by regressions that only involve matrix multiplication, the whole registration process can be computed in real time.

Forest Classification. The classification consists of two steps: First, each tree traversal of the target projection image yields a neighborhood set of training projection images that visit the same leaf node. For 100 trees the method computes the most frequently visited training projection image from the 100 neighborhood sets. Second, the method assigns the target projection image the same partition as its most nearest training neighbor's.

Regression Estimation. With the training partition $\mathcal{L}^*$ classified the method uses the learned linear regression $\mathbf{W}_{\mathcal{L}^*}^i$ of that training partition to estimate the deformation parameter c_{target}^i from the target projection intensities $\mathbf{P}_{target}$:

$$c_{target}^i = \mathbf{P}_{target} \cdot \mathbf{W}_{\mathcal{L}^*}^i.$$

3 Results

The local regression method has been validated on 500 synthetic treatment-time deformations and 5 real treatment-time deformations sampled from 5 lung datasets (pt1 to pt5). In the synthetic tests, target projection images are the DRRs computed from the Fréchet mean image warped by random treatment-time deformations sampled from the patient's deformation eigenmode space within ±3 standard deviations of the weights observed in the patient's RCCTs. Having the ground truths of the deformation parameters, the synthetic tests are used to analyze the optimal training settings (e.g., the number of training samples and partitions) in terms of the method's registration accuracy and efficiency. Moreover, to better understand the importance of the local regression, the accuracy of the forest classification and the accuracy of the local regression are also compared in this section.

3.1 The Datasets

Five lung datasets have been tested for this local regression method. Each dataset consists of 10 treatment-planning RCCTs, a target cone-beam CT (CBCT) projection (coronal-view, dimension down-sampled to 128 × 96) scanned at the patient's end-of-expiration (EE) phase, and a validating 3D EE-phase CBCT reconstructed at treatment time. As shown in Fig. 1 those five datasets represent very different pathological states and imaging fields of views (FOVs). For example, patient 1 and 4 (pt 1 and 4) have a shorter CT scan along the superior-inferior (SI) direction and therefore the simulated projections have truncations; Patient 4 has only one lung, and patient 5 has an extended view toward the abdominal region. For all five patient datasets, their target projections are all imaged in the patients' EE phases. The estimated deformations are validated by treatment-time reconstructed cone-beam CTs (CBCTs) at the same EE phases. Particularly, the results measure mean target registration errors (mTREs) as (1) the tumor centroid differences (for real tests) or (2) the average deformation differences of a lung voxel (for synthetic tests) between the estimated CTs (Fréchet mean images warped by the estimated deformations) and the validating CBCTs (for real tests) or the ground truth target CTs (for synthetic tests). Tumors are manually segmented in both CTs and CBCTs.

3.2 Synthetic Tests

For each lung dataset, 100 testing projections and testing deformation parameters are randomly sampled in the patient's deformation eigenmode space. The registration accuracy and efficiency has been tested with varying number of training samples and with varying number of partitions.

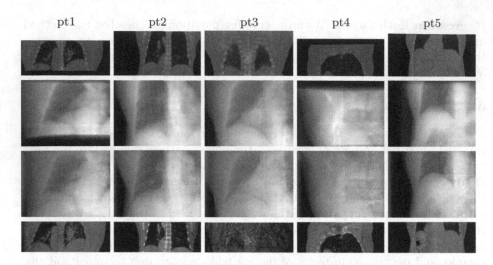

Fig. 1. The 5 lung datasets. Top row: the middle coronal slices of the patients' Fréchet mean CT images. Second row: DRRs of the Fréchet mean CT images. Third row: target projection images at the end-of-expiration (EE) phase. Fourth row: validating reconstructed cone-beam CTs (CBCTs) at the EE phases.

Training Space Sampling and Partitioning. Five different numbers of partitions have been chosen for testing: 1, 2, 4, 8, and 16 partitions. The method partitions the training samples recursively by normalized graph cuts. As shown in Fig. 2, the method first separates the training space along the first deformation eigenmode because it contributes the greatest variation of the training deformations.

Forest Classification. Also shown in Fig. 2, the decision forest successfully classify most of the testing samples into the correct training partitions. The error partition assignments only happen on the partition boundaries.

Forest Classification vs. Local Regression Accuracy. Forest classification selects a nearest training neighbor for each testing target projection image. The deformation parameters of the selected nearest neighbor can be used as an rough estimation, and the further local regression provides refinements of the forest classification. To demonstrate the refinement improvement of the local regression, 500 synthetic tests are generated from the 5 lung datasets (100 tests each). The accuracy is measured by the mean deformation error appeared in the lung. As shown in Fig. 3(a), both forest classification and the local regression accuracy have improved greatly with the increasing number of training samples. However, the accuracy of the forest classification converges to 0.5 mm where the local regression converges at 0.05 mm, which shows a 10-fold error reduction.

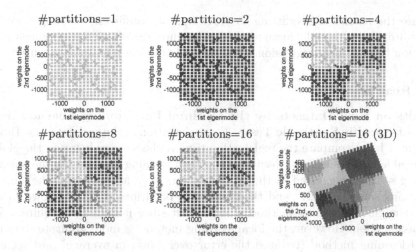

Fig. 2. Training samples partitioning and forest classification results of a lung dataset. Circular dots are 21^3 training samples in the deformation eigenmode space. Square dots are the 100 random testing samples colored by different partitions decided by the forest.

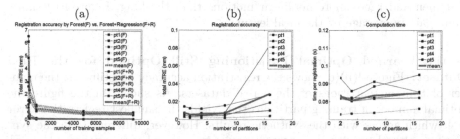

Fig. 3. (a) Average deformation errors of a lung voxel in the 100 synthetic tests for each patient with varying numbers of training samples. The registration accuracy of the forest classification (F) is compared with the accuracy of the forest classification followed by local regression (F+R). In the figures the local regression uses the optimal number of training partitions that yields the most accurate registration. (b) Average deformation errors of a lung voxel and (c) average registration time in the 100 synthetic tests for each patient with varying numbers of training partitions (2, 4, 8, and 16 partitions) for 21^3 training samples.

The More Partitions, The Better? Registration time and accuracy are investigated with the number of the training partitions used. Figures 3(b) and 4(a) show the registration error reduces and then increases with the number of training partitions. This suggests that the local regression enhances the registration accuracy if the a proper partition of the training space is applied. For the results shown in the figure, with the $N = 21^3$ training samples the linear regressions best fit to a smaller partition rather than to the entire training set. The increasing errors observed in the over-partitioning situations (the number of partitions

>8) are the results of overfitting to partitions of insufficient training samples. Figure 3(c) shows that the method yields minimum registration time (forest classification time + local regression time) when 4 training partitions are used.

3.3   Real Tests

Results on Real Datasets by the Optimal Partitioning Learned from Patient-Specific Synthetic Tests. For registration of the real datasets, Table 1 and Fig. 4(b)(c) compare the registration time and accuracy between the global and local learning methods. Results of the local learning method use the optimal training settings suggested by the synthetic tests, e.g., for patient 2, the number of training samples $= 21^3$ and the number of partitions $= 4$. As shown in the table, the global learning method is super fast since it does not require a forest classification. However, the local learning method is more accurate than the global learning method (reduced the error over 1 mm in average) and yet still can be computed in real time (70 ms per registration in average). In addition, for target projection images having more abdominal FOV like patient 5's, the great error reduction shows the method's ability to learn the nonlinear relationship between the projection intensities and the deformation parameters as the abdomen undergoes more nonlinear motions than the lung. Figure 4(b) shows 1 mm gain in average by the local learning.

Is the Learned Optimal Partitioning Still Optimal for the Real Dataset? Figure 4(b)(c) shows the registration accuracy and time vs. the number of training partitions of the 5 real datasets. As shown in the figure the optimal number of training partitions that yields the smallest registration error is 4, which agrees with the synthetic results. However, different than the synthetic results, the registration error does not increase when more than 4 training partitions are used. One possible cause for this inconsistency is that the optimal number of training partitions depends on the distribution of the target projection images in the training deformation space. For example, the synthetic target projection images are distributed in the whole training deformation space whereas the real target projection images are all in the EE phases, which lie in a region close to the boundaries of the training deformation space (see boundaries in the sub-figures in Fig. 2). Consequently, regressions fitted to a smaller training partition will tend to have better estimation of this extreme testing deformation.

Table 1. Registration time and accuracy of the five real datasets. The accuracy is measured by the tumor centroid differences between the estimated CTs and the validating CBCTs.

Global learning	pt1	pt2	pt3	pt4	pt5	Local learning	pt1	pt2	pt3	pt4	pt5
#partitions	1	1	1	1	1	#partitions	4	4	4	4	2
mTRE (mm)	4.18	1.94	3.78	2.12	6.65	mTRE (mm)	3.23	1.85	3.08	2.11	2.78
Time (s)	0.001	0.001	0.001	0.001	0.001	Time (s)	0.06	0.07	0.07	0.06	0.07

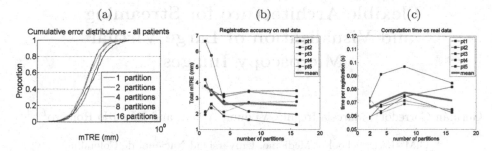

Fig. 4. (a) Cumulative error distributions on 500 synthetic tests from 5 lung datasets (21^3 training images for each dataset). (b) Registration accuracy and (c) time vs. the number of training partitions on 5 real lung datasets.

4   Conclusions and Discussion

This paper presented a novel shape-space-localized learning method for 2D/3D deformable registration and uses regression learning as an example. The method learns regression mappings in each local deformation space partitioned by normalized graph cuts. In the application stage it uses the learned regression mappings of a forest-classified partition to yield more accurate 2D/3D deformable registration than the global regression learning method. The optimal training settings obtained from the patient-specific synthetic tests can be used to help registrations achieve near-optimum accuracy and efficiency on the patient's real data. Also, the method provides a general local learning framework that could be expected to be applicable to other learning-based registration methods, i.e., learning a local distance metric for parameter interpolation in [2].

References

1. Chou, C.R., Frederick, B., Mageras, G., Chang, S., Pizer, S.: 2D/3D image registration using regression learning. Comput. Vis. Image Underst. **117**(9), 1095–1106 (2013)
2. Chou, C.-R., Pizer, S.: Real-time 2D/3D deformable registration using metric learning. In: Menze, B.H., Langs, G., Lu, L., Montillo, A., Tu, Z., Criminisi, A. (eds.) MCV 2012. LNCS, vol. 7766, pp. 1–10. Springer, Heidelberg (2013)
3. Shi, J., Malik, J.: Normalized cuts and image segmentation. IEEE Trans. Pattern Anal. Mach. Intell. **22**, 888–905 (2000)
4. Criminisi, A., Shotton, J. (eds.): Decision Forests for Computer Vision and Medical Image Analysis. Advances in Computer Vision and Pattern Recognition. Springer, London (2013)
5. Breiman, L.: Random forests. Mach. Learn. **45**(1), 5–32 (2001)

Flexible Architecture for Streaming and Visualization of Large Virtual Microscopy Images

Germán Corredor[1], Marcela Iregui[2], Viviana Arias[1], and Eduardo Romero[1](✉)

[1] CIM@LAB, School of Medicine, Universidad Nacional de Colombia,
Carrera 45 No 26-85, Bogotá, Colombia
{gcorredorp,vlariasp,edromero}@unal.edu.co
[2] Acceder Research Group, School of Engineering,
Universidad Militar Nueva Granada, Carrera 11 No 101-80, Bogotá, Colombia
hilda.iregui@unimilitar.edu.co

Abstract. The growing interest in visualization and interaction with large data has brought out the development of strategies that speed up data availability. Applications such as Virtual Microscopy are requiring efficacious, efficient and ubiquitous strategies to access very large images. Current navigation approaches use a JPEG pyramidal structure to stream and visualize very large images, a strategy that demands an important computational infrastructure and a complex management of the multiple files that compose the pyramid. This article introduces a novel JPEG2000-based service oriented architecture for streaming and visualizing very large images under scalable strategies. Results suggest that the proposed architecture facilitates transmission and visualization of large images, while it efficiently uses the available device resources.

Keywords: Browsing · JPEG2000 · Mega images · Streaming · Visualization · Virtual microscopy · Web services

1 Introduction

Virtual Microscopy (VM) is a pathology subdiscipline that aims to store virtual slides to be examined at any time. Typically, a histopathological specimen is digitized at the higher possible magnification to provide the pathologist with a maximum amount of information. For this reason, sizes of virtual microscopy images are typically on the order of hundreds of megabytes and therefore long loading times are required to open and display such files. An optimal interaction with such large data volumes depends on the type of stitching strategy to assembly the virtual slide and the particular method to code, store and display a specific Region of Interest (RoI). In spite of the availability of very rapid motorized microscopes, the virtual microscopy has remained reduced to some research scenarios, among others due to the lack of adapted visualization and navigation strategies.

B. Menze et al. (Eds.): MCV 2013, LNCS 8331, pp. 34–43, 2014.
DOI: 10.1007/978-3-319-05530-5_4, © Springer International Publishing Switzerland 2014

Usually, images are captured, stitched and arranged using pyramidal structures that facilitate availability of different image resolutions for a particular request [7]. A RoI Deployment requires the composition of a mosaic of images in formats such as JPEG, GIF or BMP, devised for storing but not for interacting, as required in virtual microscopy [3]. Moreover, such image composition demands a large number of files to be constantly uploading and downloading from memory [7], constituting an expensive framework that wastes important machine resources. A well-known application that uses the pyramidal strategy is Google Earth, which allows display and visualization of large satellite images. Google Earth has been tested for virtual microscopy images [7], reporting the authors a pleasant interaction experience when navigating a single image on a conventional computer. However, if a whole virtual slide must be examined, it is necessary to export a large number of files to generate the required pyramidal structure, an issue that may be aggravated if the navigation is performed on a set of slides. Commercial available software [9] allows to pan and zoom in and out virtual slides, yet this system is computationally very demanding and requires a powerful infrastructure, v.g., experiments performed by our pathologist found that the stand alone application interacts with three images but ten images blocked a standard computer (2.8 Ghz quad-core processor and 5 GB RAM memory). In contrast, the JPEG2000 (J2K) standard, devised to deal with different navigation scenarios, is entailed with a natural multiscale representation, which in addition is granular and flexible [8]. A J2K image consists of modular data containers, able to support the independent reconstruction of regions of interest [4]. This standard allows progressive transmission and random access, permitting to stream and visualize specific spatial regions at any desired resolution level and quality. These statements reinforce the idea that this standard is flexible enough as to support and visualize large virtual microscopy images [3], case in which a progressive data transmission is the basic condition to cope with different types of clients that simultaneously might be accessing the same set of virtual slides.

This work introduces a service oriented architecture that exploits the JPEG2000 paradigm to remotely interact with a database of Virtual Slides via web services. The proposed model allows to optimize the microscopy workflow in several ways: 1. Using a single file to cope with the different requests at any scale, random spatial access or desired quality; 2. Achieving a selective transmission through the net by decoding specifically the data associated to a particular request and thereby optimizing the bandwidth use; 3. Visualizing RoIs that accurately meet the user requirements at any time of the navigation process; 4. Allowing lossless decodification, an important requirement for medical imaging applications since there are concerns about potential large errors being introduced by lossy compression; 5. Decoding at the client side; and 6. simultaneously interacting with a large number of VS by displaying the smaller VS magnification. The results demonstrate how the JPEG2000 based architecture offers a proper structure to manage information at different scales, random locations and qualities, using a single file, in contrast to the complex topology required to deal with thousands of compressed JPEG files in case of the pyramidal representation. Furthermore, the resource usage is efficient, offering proper response times and allowing to deploy and interact with several images without requiring an expensive infrastructure.

The paper is organized as follows. In Sect. 2, it is introduced the proposed model for streaming and visualization of large virtual microscopy images, including an overview of the J2K and JPIP standards. Section 3 presents experimental results providing evidence the performance and efficacy of the model. Finally, Sect. 4 features a brief conclusions.

2   Methodology

2.1   Representation of Images

A single J2K data stream typically contains numerous embedded subsets, which stand for a large number of different spatial resolutions, image quality layers and spatial regions. This multidimensional access to data is defined in the J2K standard as spatially adjacent code-blocks, named precincts. Each precinct is represented as a collection of packets, each packet associated to a particular quality layer, resolution level and color component. These embedded compressed data subsets represent a particular portion of visual information that can be incrementally improved by adding the missing elements [5]. Therefore, a query at a particular spatial region, resolution or quality can be retrieved from the specific packets in the bitstream.

While a J2K codestream provides a number of mechanisms for locating and extracting portions of the compressed image data for any purpose, namely, retransmission, storage, display, or editing, the compression standard itself describes only a codestream syntax, suitable for storing the compressed data within a single file [1]. For this reason, communication is handled via web services using a JPIP-based protocol, which provides a network protocol that allows for the interactive and progressive transmission of the J2K coded data from a server to a client, i.e, only the requested portions of an image are processed [2].

2.2   System Architecture

The proposed architecture exploits the JPEG2000 granularity by splitting the main tasks of the data processing into three layers. The architecture and their main components are shown in Fig. 1.

Storage Layer. This layer is the repository of the compressed images and their respective indexes. Each J2K image is stored in a single file. Besides, customized index files are used to speed up a random access to specific portions of the image codestream; the use of such files is recommended in the JPIP standard specification [2]. The index files provide an organized structure containing the image data (dimensions, number of resolution levels, number of quality layers, etc.) and the byte ranges of the main header as well as each image packet to

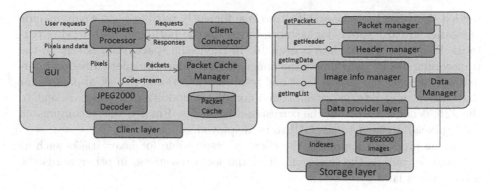

Fig. 1. Top-level runtime view of the architecture.

facilitate identification and extraction of bytes from the J2K files. Index tracking, request scalability w.r.t. to the index file size and performance are facilitated by storing the image index in multiple small-size files so that only the required index file is loaded in memory.

Data Provider Layer. This layer is responsible for any interaction with the storage layer and provides the services to allow the client to access the Virtual Slide. The services provided by this layer deal with each request independently, thereby guaranteeing a simultaneous information access.

This layer provides services with four main methods. The first delivers a list of the images available to be accessed. The second receives the name of one of the available images and delivers information such as dimensions, number of resolution levels, number of quality layers, among others. The third method also receives the name of certain image, but it delivers the bytes of the main image header, which is extracted from the compressed file, necessary to perform the decoding task. Finally, the fourth method receives a list of packet indexes of certain image and delivers the corresponding bytes for the requested packets, also extracted from the J2K file.

Client Layer. This layer communicates with the services provided by the logic layer and is responsible for the access and interaction with the Virtual Slides. The client is composed of several modules that allow a user to set the image regions to be streamed and visualized.

The client receives the query, containing particular coordinates, resolution level and quality percentage associated to the requested region from a graphic interface. When an expert is navigating, it is possible that a requested region will be needed in the future so that a cache policy is implemented by storing the received packets or tiles from the server, and retrieving them if needed (the cache memory size is a device dependent parameter). Currently, this module uses the LRU (least recently used) policy to discard packets and free memory, if needed. Nevertheless, the architecture is sufficiently flexible as to easily include any other discard policy, for instance based on the pathologist's browsing patterns. When a required data is available in the cache space, data is sent to the transcoding library, which uses the image main header, the queried region information (dimensions, quality layer and resolution level) and the set of packets for that region, and returns a transcoded compliant codestream, which is sent to the J2K decoder to obtain the corresponding pixels. Finally, the uncompressed data (pixels) are sent to the GUI to be displayed.

In the proposed approach, the client is responsible for heavy tasks such as decoding as well as the management of the local resources, in other words the server side is lazy.

3   Experimentation

3.1   Experimental Setup

Validation of the proposed model was performed by implementing the proposed architecture: the storage and data provider layers were deployed on a computer with 4 GB RAM memory and a 2.4 GHz quad core processor. The application was developed on the Java EE 1.5 platform. The GlassFish Application Server was used to deploy the application and to publish the web services.

The client application was developed in the Java platform and tests were performed on a computer with 4 GB RAM memory and 2.71 GHz dual core processor. Decoding was performed using the JasPer library [6] through the Java Native Interface.

3.2   Dataset

Experiments were performed with a dataset consisting of twenty skin biopsies of patients, diagnosed with different types of basal cell carcinoma, embedded in paraffin and stained with Hematoxylin-Eosin. The set of histological samples was provided by the Pathology Department of the Universidad Nacional de Colombia and is representative of what pathologists usually observe in their clinical routine. The image resolutions vary from 104 to 340 mega pixels, and their sizes range between 630 MB and 972 MB.

The images were J2K compressed by generating a codestream stored in a extensionless single file. The images were coded using the following parameters, which were appropriate for the study but they are not restrictive: Lossless filter (W5x3), 4 decomposition levels (5 resolutions) and 10 quality layers. In addition, the images were spatially split into JPEG2000 precincts with sizes of 32×32 (for the image at the lowest resolution), 64×64, 128×128, 256×256 and 512×512 (for the highest resolution image).

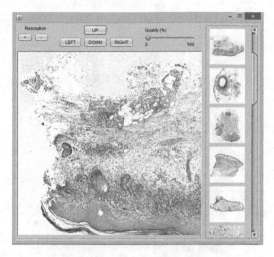

Fig. 2. Screenshot of the custom graphic interface to interact with the image dataset. At the top of the user interface there are the UI controls to interact with the image, displayed below; these controls perform the panning, zoom and quality refinement operations. The right side panel shows the list of available images for interaction.

3.3 Experimentation

The performance of the proposed architecture was validated by measuring the response times of the client side for a series of requests performed by a pathologist during a real navigation, using a custom graphic user interface (Fig. 2), which presents to the expert the whole list of available virtual slides in the database. The scene was divided to include in a central panel the slide under examination and the set of slides at the right. The pathologist interacted with the whole dataset and performed several panning, zoom and quality refinement operations, using a 3 G network. Figure 3 shows the pathologist's browsing protocol when accessing an image for diagnosis purposes.

3.4 Experimental Results

During such microscopical exploration, the transmission spanning time over the network was measured, that is to say, the time spent since the client sends a request and receives a response from the web services. Transmission time was measured for each pathologist request. Figure 4 shows the transmission times for the more representative images (the ones that were deeply examined by the pathologist). It can be seen that transmission times, in general, are low; they are not exceeding 450 ms when transmitting the whole RoI, a time required for uploading the first window of the navigation. During actual navigations, this time drastically reduced since a new request is usually a 20 % of the precedent frame. Transmission times were variable because the amount of information being streamed is dependent on the particular image, on the particular requested

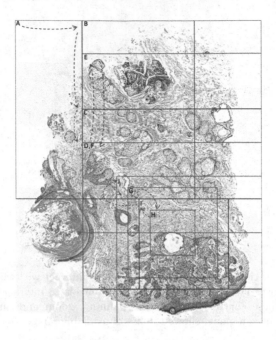

Fig. 3. Browsing protocol of a pathologist when accessing a sample image for diagnosis purposes. Frames A-F represent regions requested during panning operations. Frames G-H represent regions requested during zoom-in operations. Frame H includes operations of manual quality refinement. Finally, frames I-J represent regions requested during zoom-out operations.

data and the cached data. In general, the first navigation image requires more data because a larger image area is being visualized at the lowest resolution level. The following requests usually take less time since the application uses the cached packets for magnification and panning operations. As expected, the quality refinement operation requires higher times (for example request 11 for the image Imghistopat-13), however it is not a common process.

In the proposed approach, the client is responsible for the decoding process, a demanding task in computational terms because of the J2K complexity. Most of the available decoders are not really granular and they allow just compression-decompression operations. The strategy adopted here was then to modify the requested parameters in resolution, RoI or quality, at the level of the JPEG2000 image main header so that with any available decoder gives a selective decoding. Decoding times were measured for each pathologist request. Figure 5 shows the decoding times for each requested region during the browsing protocol. Results show that decoding times remains low, below the 300 ms.

The previous results demonstrate a proper system performance. It is responding in less than a second per request, which, according to the pathologist, is appropriate for diagnosis and training tasks in virtual microscopy scenarios.

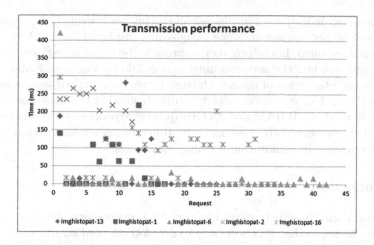

Fig. 4. Transmission time for each pathologist's request during the browsing of the more relevant images.

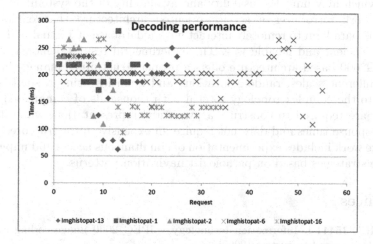

Fig. 5. Decoding time for each pathologist's request during the browsing of the more relevant images.

Furthermore, the system allows the pathologists to naturally shift from visualizing one image to another: just by clicking over the virtual slide thumbnail (image at the lowest magnification level) in the right panel of the GUI (Fig. 2); this is a clear advantage over optical microscopes since there is no need to remove the physical slide being examined, to set the new one and to adjust the lenses to proper visualization. The Pathologist pointed out that visualization of the lower magnification is crucial in terms of usability and interaction since it allows an expert to simultaneously examine a set of cases and to retrieve relevant information connected with the case displayed in the central panel.

Furthermore, in despite of displaying all the images (twenty), the application performance is not impacted, since images are displayed in short times and interaction is seamless. In the proposed approach, the client is responsible for the decoding process, i.e., the server is only responsible for extracting and sending data, allowing interaction of users with large image datasets without requiring a very powerful and/or expensive infrastructure. Instead of the basic/low features of the server used (4 GB RAM and 2.4 GHz quad core processor), this experiment shows that the presented architecture is suitable for interaction with large virtual microscopy images in exploration and diagnosis tasks.

4   Conclusions

Visualization and interaction of large virtual microscopy images are very demanding tasks, so that it is necessary to develop adapted strategies that meet user requests and palliate limitations of visualization devices. Some commercial applications require to deal with a complex organization and hierarchy of files and demand a high computational capacity to allow users interact with large images, which may limit the usability and availability of the system.

This work introduces a service oriented architecture that exploits the JPEG2000 paradigm to remotely interact with a database of Virtual Slides in an effective, efficient and flexible way. The experimental results demonstrate how the JPEG2000 based architecture offers a proper structure to manage information at different scales, random locations and qualities using a single file, in contrast to the complex topology to deal with thousands of compressed JPEG files that are required to construct a pyramidal representation, while it offers proper response times and does not require an expensive infrastructure.

Future work includes experimentation of simultaneous access and implementing cache strategies based on pathologist navigation patterns.

References

1. ISO/IEC 15444-1. Information technology - JPEG 2000 image coding system - Part 1: Core coding system (2000)
2. ISO/IEC 15444-9. Information technology - JPEG 2000 image coding system - Part 9: Interactivity tools, APIs and protocols (2004)
3. Iregui, M., Gómez, F., Romero, E.: Strategies for efficient virtual microscopy in pathological samples using JPEG2000. Micron. **38**, 700–713 (2007)
4. Rosenbaum, R., Schumann, H.: JPEG2000-based viewer guidance for mobile image browsing. In: 12th International Multi-Media Modelling Conference Proceedings. Beijing, China (2006)
5. Taubman, D.: Remote browsing of JPEG2000 images. In: Proceedings IEEE ICIP, Rochester, USA (2002)
6. Adams, M.D., Kossentini F.: Jasper - a software-based jpeg-2000 codec implementation. http://www.ece.uvic.ca/frodo/jasper
7. Alfaro, L., et al.: Compatability of virtual microscopy equipment: an analysis of different panoramic image software. Rev Esp Patol. (2011). doi:10.1016/j.patol.2011.01.009

8. Skodras, A., Christopoulos, C., Ebrahimi, T.: The JPEG 2000 still image compression standard. IEEE Sig. Process. Mag. **18**(5), 36–58 (2001)
9. Aperio Technologies Inc.: Aperio Image Analysis. http://tmalab.jhmi.edu/aperiou/userguides/Image_Analysis_UG.pdf&gt

2D-PCA Shape Models: Application to 3D Reconstruction of the Human Teeth from a Single Image

Aly S. Abdelrehim[1(✉)], Aly A. Farag[1], Ahmed M. Shalaby[1],
and Moumen T. El-Melegy[2]

[1] Computer Vision and Image Processing Laboratory, University of Louisville,
Louisville, KY 40292, USA
aly_saber@yahoo.com
[2] Electrical Engineering Department, Assiut University, Assiut 71516, Egypt

Abstract. Accurate modeling of human teeth is mandatory for many reasons. Some of them are (1) Providing comfort to patients during mold process, and (2) Enhancing the accuracy level for oral orthodontist and dental care personnel. Shape from Shading (SFS) proved to be of great help in this problem, considering the fact that human tooth surface is textureless. In this paper, we address the problem of 3D tooth reconstruction, and improve the current algorithms. The approached developed in this paper reconstructs the teeth from single image shading with 2D-PCA shape priors that have more sophisticated reflectance model. Oren-Nayar-Wolff model was used for modeling the surface reflectance. This formulation uses shape priors as got from a set of training CT scans of real human teeth. Our experiments show promising quantitative results, which builds the infrastructure for having an optical based approach that accounts for inexpensive and radiationless human tooth reconstruction.

1 Introduction

Accurate 3D representation of the teeth and the jaw is mandatory for many dental and maxillofacial surgery applications such as endodontic procedures, treatment of malocclusion problems and treatment simulations. conventional physical solid models have many drawbacks that are not present in 3D CAD models such as the bulky size, that gets financial and logistic problems. Since multi-image reconstruction techniques do not account much on texture information, SFS algorithms are significant in human teeth reconstruction introducing many advantages such as low cost, providing accurate representation of the tooth crowns, and the minimal use of cameras as only one is used within the cramped confines of the mouth [1,2,12].

The two systems that showed most promise in the last few years are the iTero (Cadance) and Lava. The probes in both systems are bulky and requiring multiple scans to get full coverage of the oral cavity. The Lava system requires the use of a visible powder to get good registration, and has problems with

B. Menze et al. (Eds.): MCV 2013, LNCS 8331, pp. 44–52, 2014.
DOI: 10.1007/978-3-319-05530-5_5, © Springer International Publishing Switzerland 2014

depth of field. The iTero has a heavier probe and can only capture one tooth at a time, requiring five views of each tooth. Blood and saliva causes additional inaccuracies with both systems.

There has been a substantial amount of work regarding 3D reconstruction of human teeth using intraoral camera and SFS techniques. Abdelrahim et al. [1] proposed an image-based 3D reconstruction of the human jaw using shape from shading that benefit from the camera parameters. They assumed the tooth surface to have Lambertian reflectance and the light source to be a single point source at infinity. Unfortunately, such assumptions are no longer held in case of intraoral imaging environment for human teeth. Also, their work did not give any quantitative results.

Recently, Abelrahim et al. [2] presented a 3D reconstruction of the human teeth using SFS with shape priors. This work is lacking in the following aspects: (1) they assumed Oren-Nayar model for tooth surface reflectance. Nonetheless, tooth surface is rough and wet. (2) Shape prior information was constructing using Principal Component Analysis where PCA is time consuming to determine the corresponding eigenvectors.

In this paper, we target further improvement in the accuracy of the human tooth reconstruction approach in [2]. Our contribution here are two-fold. First, the 2D-PCA is used to build the shape priors instead of the conventional PCA. The 2D-PCA offers two important advantages [13]: It is easier to evaluate the covariance matrix accurately since its size is much smaller. In addition, less time is required to determine the corresponding eigenvectors [13]. Second, the modified Oren-Nayar-Wolff reflectance model [11] is presumed in place of the Oren-Nayar model assumed in [2], where teeth surface is rough and wet, giving rise to Fresnel reflection due to different refractive indices of the saliva and the tooth material. The tooth surface roughness is physically measured using an optical surface profiler.

The rest of the paper is organized as follows. In Sect. 2, we explain how to build the priors shape model using 2D-PCA. In Sect. 3, image irradiance equation is briefly explained and we demonstrate how to integrate the tooth shape priors into SFS-framework. Experimental results are presented in Sect. 4, and the paper is concluded in Sect. 5.

2   Method

2.1   Data Preprocessing

The triangular meshes of the training ensemble are obtained from a high resolution computer tomography scan of human invitro teeth. A Cone-beam CT (KODAK 9000 3D Extraoral) scanner at a resolution of 0.2 × 0.2 × 0.2 mm is then used to scan the wax and teeth. where we use the Expectation-Maximization (EM) algorithm for segmentation [4]. The first surface of the training set is used as the reference to which the remaining surfaces are aligned. 3D surfaces for each tooth type are rigidly aligned to the reference using an ICP-based rigid registration algorithm [6] using the Hausdorff distance between corresponding points.

2.2 Shape Model Construction

In this paper, shape reconstruction, using 2D-PCA, is done using the height map[1] in order to extract the most significant information of training images. Unlike the conventional PCA, 2D-PCA as the name implies will have matrix information rather than vector information which means that there is no need to get image pre-transformed into a vector, let more coefficients will be needed to represent the image [13]. This needs incorporation of the conventional PCA in a further step to reduce the dimensionality of principle component matrix of 2D-PCA.

Now, let the training set consist of M training height maps $\{U_1, \ldots, U_M\}$ with size $n \times m$. All images are pre-aligned. As in [13], we obtain the mean of the training shapes, $\overline{U}$, as the average of these M height maps. To extract the shape variabilities, $\overline{U}$ is subtracted from each of the training height maps. The obtained mean-offset functions can be represented as $\{\widehat{U}_1, \ldots, \widehat{U}_M\}$. These new functions are used to measure the variabilities of the training images. We use M training teeth (for each type) images with 100×100 pixels in our experiment. According to [13], we use the M mean-offset height maps to construct the covariance matrix $\mathbf{G}$, as following:

$$\mathbf{G} = \frac{1}{M} \sum_{i=1}^{M} \widehat{U}_i^t \widehat{U}_i. \tag{1}$$

The goal of 2D-PCA is to find the optimal K eigenvectors of $\mathbf{G}$ corresponding to the largest K eigenvalues. The value of K helps to capture the necessary shape variation with minimum information. Experimentally, we find that the minimum suitable value is $K = 10$. After we choosing the eigenvectors corresponding to the 10 largest eigenvalues ($\mathbf{B} = \mathbf{b_1}, \mathbf{b_2}, \ldots, \mathbf{b_{10}}$), we obtained the principle component matrix $\mathbf{Y}_i (m = 100 \times K = 10)$ for each height map of our training set ($i = 1, 2, \ldots, M$), where $\mathbf{Y}_i = U_i \mathbf{B}^t$. For more dimensional reduction, the conventional PCA is applied on the principle components $\{\overrightarrow{\mathbf{Y}_1}, \ldots, \overrightarrow{\mathbf{Y}_M}\}$. It should be noted that, $\overrightarrow{\mathbf{Y}}$ is the vector representation of $\mathbf{Y}$. The reconstructed components (after retransforming to matrix representation) will be:

$$\widetilde{\mathbf{Y}}_{\{l,\mathbf{h}\}} = \mathbf{De}_{\{l,\mathbf{h}\}}, \tag{2}$$

where $\mathbf{D}$ is the matrix which contains L eigenvectors corresponding to L largest eigenvalues $\lambda_l, (l = 1, 2, \ldots, L)$, and $e_{\{l,h\}}$ is the set of model parameters which can be described as:

$$\mathbf{e}_{\{l,\mathbf{h}\}} = h\sqrt{\lambda_l} \tag{3}$$

where $l = \{1, \ldots, L\}$, $h = \{-\mu, \ldots \mu, \}$, and μ is a constant which can be chosen arbitrarily. The new principle components of training height maps are represented as $\{\widetilde{\mathbf{Y}}_1, \ldots, \widetilde{\mathbf{Y}}_\mathbf{N}\}$ instead of $\{\mathbf{Y}_1, \ldots, \mathbf{Y}_M\}$ where N is a constant which can be chosen arbitrarily.

---

[1] A height map is a raster image used to store values, such as surface elevation data (The depth in our case).

Given the set $\{\widetilde{\mathbf{Y}}_1, \ldots, \widetilde{\mathbf{Y}}_N\}$, the new projected training height maps are obtained as:

$$\widetilde{\mathbf{U}}_n = \widetilde{\mathbf{Y}}_n \mathbf{B}^t, \quad n = 1, 2, \ldots, N. \tag{4}$$

The shape model is required to capture the variations in the training set. This model is considered to be a weighted sum of the projected height maps (4) as:

$$u(\mathbf{x}) = \bar{\mathbf{U}} + \sum_{n=1}^{N} w_n \widetilde{\mathbf{U}}_n, \tag{5}$$

where $\bar{\mathbf{U}}$ is the mean height map (mean tooth shape), $\widetilde{\mathbf{U}}_n$ is the nth orthogonal mode of variation in the shape (also called *eigenteeth*), and $\mathbf{w} = \{w_n\}$ is called the vector of eigen coefficients or the shape vector. Only N principal components are considered in the sum, where N should be chosen large enough to be able to capture the prominent shape variations present in the human teeth.

We propose to use the function given in (5) as our explicit representation of teeth shape. Therefore, by varying $\mathbf{w}$, we vary $u(\mathbf{x})$.

3   Shape from Shading with Shape Priors

One good model for tooth surface reflectance is the Oren-Nayar-Wolff models which work well for the retro-reflection case [10]. The microscopic view of the occlusal surface height variations which proves that micro-facet reflectance models are suitable for the tooth surface. When the object is illuminated in the viewing direction, taking into account the illumination attenuation term $(1/r^2)$, the expression of the image irradiance $R(.)$ using Oren-Nayar-Wolff model can be simplified to [11]:

$$R(u(\mathbf{x})) = \frac{A(1 - F(\theta, \zeta))^2 \cos\theta + B \sin^2\theta}{r^2};$$

$$\text{s.t. } A = 1 - 0.5 \frac{\sigma^2}{\sigma^2 + 0.33}, B = 0.45 \frac{\sigma^2}{\sigma^2 + 0.09}, \tag{6}$$

where the parameter σ denotes the standard deviation of the Gaussian distribution which is used as a measure of the surface roughness, θ is the viewer/source inclination angle and F refers to the Fresnel reflection function [11] with refractive index of ζ.

From the definitions of the perspective camera as in [2], We can write $\cos\theta$ as:

$$\cos\theta = \frac{f}{\sqrt{x^2 + y^2 + f^2}} u(\mathbf{x}), \tag{7}$$

Assume the camera is modelled with a perspective projection. According to our data acquisition setup, the light source is located at the optical center. The surface is represented by [8,9]: $\mathcal{S} = \{S(\mathbf{x})/\mathbf{x} \in \Omega\}$, where $S(\mathbf{x}) = \frac{f\, u(\mathbf{x})}{\sqrt{|\mathbf{x}|^2 + f^2}}(\mathbf{x}, -f)$, with f is the camera's focal length.

In this phase, the prior shape model is embedded in SFS framework to guide the solution. The Oren-Nayar-Wolff diffuse reflection model with a near light source and perspective camera is considered.

Before the construction step, alignment is needed between the input brightness image and the reference height map. A 2D rigid image registration technique with maximization of mutual information [7] is conducted to achieve the alignment. The Oren-Nayar-Wolff model is applied for reflectance with a camera that obeys perspective projection and a light source is located at the cameras optical center. Intensity of the light is attenuated with squared distance. The idea here is to solve for the height map $u(\mathbf{x})$ that minimizes the energy functional

$$\varepsilon = \int_\Omega (I(\mathbf{x}) - R(u(\mathbf{x}))^2 d\mathbf{x}, \tag{8}$$

where $\Omega \in \Re^2$ represents the image spatial domain, and I is the image intensity.

A great advantage of the above optimization problem (8) is that the solution search space is shrunk into a finite number (N) of weights. Our goal here is to find the solution:

$$\hat{w}_n = \arg\min_{w_n} \varepsilon, n = 1, \cdots, N, \tag{9}$$

Gradient descent optimization is used for computing w_n as follows:

$$\frac{\partial w_n}{\partial t} = -\eta \frac{\partial \varepsilon}{\partial w_n}, \tag{10}$$

where η is real positive learning constant. The gradient will be as follows:

$$\frac{\partial \varepsilon}{\partial w_n} = \int_\Omega 2\left[I(\mathbf{x}) - R(u(\mathbf{x}))\right] \left(-\frac{\partial R(u(\mathbf{x}))}{\partial w_n}\right) d\mathbf{x}. \tag{11}$$

Figure 1 summarize the whole framework of the proposed method.

4   Experimental Results

To evaluate the performance of our 3D reconstruction method, we apply our approach on real human teeth. Premolar model, Mandibular molar, Mandibular third molar, Maxillary molar, and maxillary deciduous models are constructed from $30, 30, 100, 40,$ and 30 teeth respectively. The shape priors are trained using out-of-training samples (we are used 2/3 for the training and 1/3 for the test) with instances using the CT-scan of the respective teeth. The accuracy of the tooth reconstruction is assessed by comparing it to the 3D ground-truth surface as obtained from CT scan. We evaluate our algorithm (A) with two algorithms. The first algorithm (B) [2] is more recent. It is a SFS algorithm that reconstructs 3D shape of the human teeth based on the shape priors that are built using conventional PCA. The other algorithm (C) [5] is a conventional SFS approach based on the work of Ahmed et al. in [3].

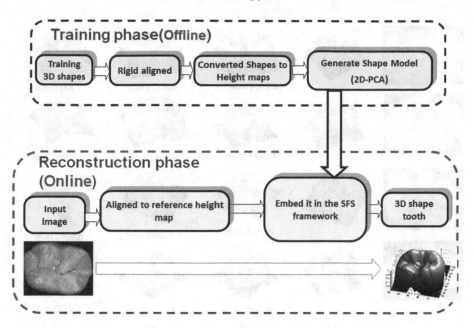

Fig. 1. The proposed 3D reconstruction of the human teeth using SFS and shape priors.

Table 1. Summary of Approaches Under Experimental Comparison. All algorithm are a perspective camera projection and the light source at the camera optical center.

	Reflectance	Priors	Reference
A	Oren-Nayar-Wolff	2D-PCA	*Proposed*
B	Oren-Nayar	PCA	[2]
C	Oren-Nayar	no	[5]

Table 1 summarizes the key differences between our proposed algorithm (A) and the others algorithms (B and C).

Figure 2 illustrated samples results from the three approaches under evaluation. Figure 2(a) demonstrates the 2D input images for different teeth models (e.g. mandibular molar, mandibular third molar, maxillary molar, and maxillary deciduous). Figure 2(b) shows the corresponding ground-truth (GT) as obtained from CT scans. Figure 2(c) shows the results of our proposed method. Figure 2(d) shows the 3D reconstruction of the human teeth using algorithm (B) while the 3D reconstruction using the traditional well-known SFS in Fig. 2(e). Clearly, better construction is provided by our proposed method. The root-mean-square (RMS) error is measured between the reconstruction surface and the GT after performing the 3D rigid registration.

The average teeth reconstruction accuracy (RMS) in mm for algorithms A, B, and C is compared for various tooth types in Table 2. It is clear that our proposed algorithm (A) outperforms the other algorithms. It is worth-mentioning that

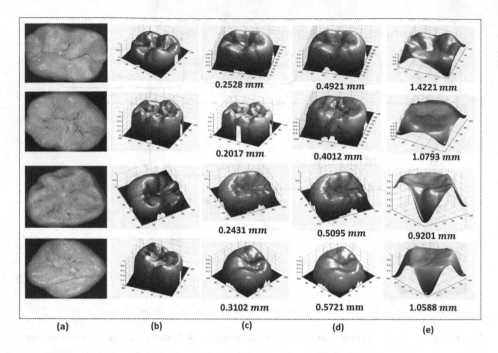

Fig. 2. Tooth reconstruction from three different algorithms. (a) 2D-image captured by the intra-oral camera.(b) GT occlusal surface generated from a CT scan of the tooth. (c) 3D Reconstruction of the human teeth using our proposed method. (d) Reconstruction using algorithm B. (e) Reconstruction using algorithm C (well-known SFS method). Beneath each reconstruction is the root-mean-square (RMS) error.

Table 2. Average teeth surface reconstruction accuracy (RMS) in mm.

Tooth Type	Proposed (A)	Algorithm (B) [2]	SFS (C) [5]
Premolar	**0.2872**	0.6502	1.3739
Mandibular molar	**0.3017**	0.6825	1.1098
Mandibular third molar	**0.2058**	0.5625	1.0702
Maxillary molar	**0.3288**	0.6646	1.2738
Maxillary deciduous	**0.2591**	0.5711	1.4317

throughout our experimentations our proposed method is faster than algorithm (B). The CPU timing is computed on a PC with Core i7 CPU@ 2.2 GHz processor and 4 GB RAM. The average time for the proposed method is 40 s. while the other algorithm (B) is 80 s.

To further demonstrate the gain out of the shape priors, another experiment is performed on real human teeth with fillings that cover significant parts of the teeth and the enamel is removed, see Fig. 3 shows the corresponding surface reconstructions by our proposed approach. Note that the teeth are successfully and completely reconstructed, in spite of the tooth filling regions with different

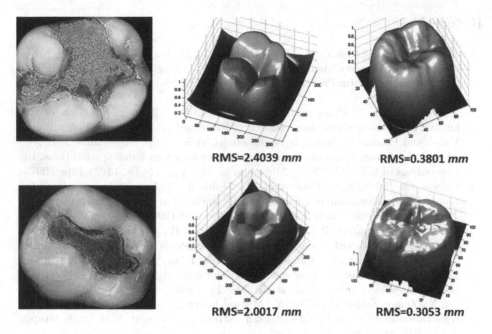

Fig. 3. Experiment on teeth with significant fillings. Input test image shown in the first column. The second column illustrated reconstruction by the traditional SFS without shape priors. Third column shown the proposed algorithm. Beneath each reconstruction is the root-mean-square (RMS) error.

colors and albedo characteristics in the input images. This notable outcome of the proposed approach becomes more evident when compared to the tooth reconstruction by Algorithm used SFS without shape priors.

5   Conclusion

In this paper, we have proposed a 3D reconstruction of human tooth models from optical imagery using shape from shading with 2D-PCA shape priors. The proposed method improves the 3D reconstruction of the human teeth by incorporating more-sophisticated reflectance models. In dental application improvements are considered significant even if the improvement is a fraction of millimeter. We used the Oren-Nayar-Wolff reflectance model which is a physically deep model for diffuse reflectance from shiny but slightly rough surfaces. Our results are preferred to other approaches in the literature since fine teeth details can be reconstructed and the resulting surface is more realistic. Also the execution time is reasonable and practical in the sense of applying the proposed system in clinic. Another major difference in our approach, the output file of our approach will be readily available as an STL file instead of locked in a proprietary format such as commercial systems have done.

References

1. Abdelrahim, A., Abdelrahman, M., Abdelmunim, H., Farag, A., Miller, M.: Novel image-based 3D reconstruction of the human jaw using shape from shading and feature descriptors. In: Proceedings of the British Machine Vision Conference, pp. 41.1–41.11 (2011)
2. Abdelrahim, A., El-Melegy, M., Farag, A.: Realistic 3D reconstruction of the human teeth using shape from shading with shape priors. In: IEEE Computer Vision and Pattern Recognition Workshops (CVPRW), pp. 64–69, June 2012
3. Ahmed, A., Farag, A.: Shape from shading under various imaging conditions. In: Proceedings of IEEE CVPR'07, Minneapolis, MN, pp. X1–X8, 18–23 June 2007
4. Carson, C., Belongie, S., Greenspan, H., Malik, J.: Blobworld: image segmentation using expectation-maximization and its application to image querying. IEEE Trans. Pattern Anal. Mach. Intell. **24**(8), 1026–1038 (2002)
5. Carter, C.N., Pusateri, R.J., Chen, D., Ahmed, A.H., Farag, A.A.: Shape from shading for hybrid surfaces as applied to tooth reconstruction. In: International Conference on Image Processing (ICIP10), Hong Kong, pp. 4049–4052 (2010)
6. Chui, H., Rangarajan, A.: A new point matching algorithm for non-rigid registration. Comput. Vis. Image Underst. **89**, 114–141 (2003)
7. Lu, X., Zhang, S., Su, H., Chen, Y.: Mutual information-based multimodal image registration using a novel joint histogram estimation. Comput. Med. Imag. Graph. **32**(3), 202–209 (2008)
8. Prados, E., Camilli, F., Faugeras, O.: A unifying and rigorous shape from shading method adapted to realistic data and applications. J. Math. Imag. Vis. **25**, 307–328 (2006)
9. Prados, E., Faugeras, O.: Shape from shading: a well-posed problem? In: IEEE CVPR 2005. vol. 2, pp. 870–877, June 2005
10. Ragheb, H., Hancock, E.: Surface radiance correction for shape from shading. Pattern Recogn. **38**, 1574–1595 (2005)
11. Wolff, L., Nayar, S., Oren, M.: Improved diffuse reflection models for computer vision. IJCV **30**(1), 55–71 (1998)
12. Yamany, S., Farag, A., Tasman, D., Farman, A.: A 3-D reconstruction system for the human jaw using a sequence of optical images. IEEE TMI **19**, 538–547 (2000)
13. Yang, J., Zhang, D., Frangi, A., Yu Yang, J.: Two-dimensional PCA: a new approach to appearance-based face representation and recognition. IEEE Trans. Pattern Anal. Mach. Intell. **26**(1), 131–137 (2004)

Class-Specific Regression Random Forest
for Accurate Extraction of Standard Planes
from 3D Echocardiography

Kiryl Chykeyuk$^{(\boxtimes)}$, Mohammad Yaqub, and J. Alison Noble

Department of Engineering Science, Institute of Biomedical Engineering,
University of Oxford, Oxford, UK
kiryl.chykeyuk@eng.ox.ac.uk

Abstract. This paper proposes a class-specific regression random forest as a fully automatic algorithm for extraction of the standard view planes from 3D echocardiography. We present a natural, continuous parameterization of the plane detection task and address it by the regression voting algorithm. We integrate the voxel class label information into the training of the regression forest to exclude irrelevant classes from voting. This yields a class-specific regression forest. Two objective functions are employed to optimize for both the class label and the class-conditional regression parameters. During testing, high uncertainty class-specific predictors are excluded from voting, maximizing the confidence of the continuous output predictions.

The method is validated on a dataset of 25 3D echocardiographic images. Compared to the classic regression forest [1], the class-specific regression forest demonstrates a significant improvement in the accuracy of the detected planes.

Keywords: Class-specific regression random forests · Plane detection · 3D echocardiography

1   Introduction

Extraction of the standard views from 3D echocardiography plays an important role in the assessment of heart function. In clinical practice, cardiologists analyze the three standard views – 2-chamber view (2C), 3-chamber view (3C) and 4-chamber view (4C). This plane detection is done visually and is subjective, time-consuming and operator-dependent. Therefore, quick and reliable methods for automatic detection of the standard views in 3D echocardiography are pertinent towards the development of accurate assessment of heart function.

In this paper, we present a fully automatic method to extract the best 2C, 3C and 4C image planes from 3D ultrasound volumes of the left ventricle (LV) using the class-specific regression forest.

Regression forests. Regression forests [1] estimate non-linear mapping from the input space to the space of a continuous output space. In plane detection, the regression forest learns the non-linear mapping directly from voxels to the parameters of the

B. Menze et al. (Eds.): MCV 2013, LNCS 8331, pp. 53–62, 2014.
DOI: 10.1007/978-3-319-05530-5_6, © Springer International Publishing Switzerland 2014

plane. Regression forests found use in medical imaging fairly recently and first were applied in [2] for anatomy detection in CT scan of the whole body. Since then, the regression forests have been successfully applied in a few medical image analysis applications [2–6].

Class-specific regression forest. In this work, we propose to integrate voxel label information into the training of the regression forest algorithm, which yields the class-specific regression forest. This extra information allows to exclude from voting irrelevant to the problem classes. Specifically, for standard views detection from 3D echocardiographic images of the LV, information beyond the left and right ventricles does not contain any useful knowledge about the planes. However, due to their high proportion in the image, the background voxels dominate in the learning process, resulting in the low confidence predictors, and, therefore, must be excluded from the voting. In the class-specific forest, two objective functions are used to optimize for the class label and the class-conditional continuous parameters of the plane. This ensures that a single class label dominates at each leaf, and the confidence of its corresponding class-conditional parameter distribution is high. At the training stage only voxels from the myocardium and the blood pool participate in the optimization of the plane parameters. During testing, each voxel uses only one high-confidence class-conditional distribution per leaf node for prediction of the plane. Predictors from other classes are excluded from voting.

Our work takes a similar approach to that of Hough Forests in [7]. During testing, the datapoints from activated leaf nodes vote directly in the Hough accumulator space. However, the Hough forests are trained for object classification, and the votes are allowed only from the instances of the same object, whereas in our work multiple classes, i.e. myocardium and blood pool, are allowed to vote for the parameters of the plane of interest.

The main contribution of this paper is in the use of a natural, one-step approach for plane extraction from a 3D volume using regression voting. The traditional two-step detection approach, where a number of candidate planes are first extracted from the volume, followed by classification of the extracted planes, has two weaknesses: (i) the candidate selection space is extensive and the actual planes can be missed during the selection procedure (ii) during classification, only information from the candidate slice is considered, ignoring any structural information in the rest of the volume. In this work, we use a natural parameterization of the plane, which considers the whole space of possible planes. During regression, every voxel of the volume votes on the parameters of the plane, and hence, the whole 3D volume participates in the decision.

The contributions of this work are twofold. First, we address the problem of plane detection from a 3D volume using a natural regression voting approach. Secondly, we propose a class-specific regression voting procedure, where the class label information is incorporated into the training procedure to help maximize the confidence of the continuous outputs.

2   Class-Specific Regression Voting

2.1   Training

Let $\mathbf{v}$ be a voxel in a 3D volume, represented by a feature vector $f = (f_1, f_2, \ldots, f_n)$; each voxel is assigned the voxel class label c, and a distance vector $\mathbf{d} = (d_x, d_y, d_z)$ to the plane Γ. The training dataset comprises a set of uniformly sampled voxels $\{\mathbf{V}_i = (f_i, \mathbf{d}_i, c_i)\}$. The class-specific regression forest consists of a set of trees; each tree is constructed using the training dataset $\mathbf{V}$. The training starts at the root node with all available training data, Fig. 1. The data is split to the left and the right child nodes according to the node optimization criteria described below. The splitting continues until the criteria to stop are reached. Each leaf node l stores the discrete probability distribution of the class label $p(c|l)$, estimated as the proportion of voxels per class that reached the leaf, and the three-dimensional distance vectors $\mathbf{d}_c$ that

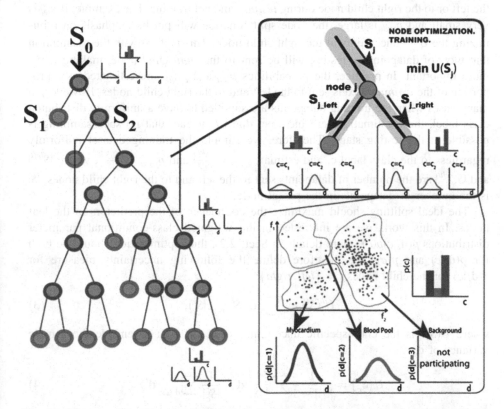

Fig. 1. Class-specific regression forest. Training. During training, the data arrived at the split node j is divided to the left and the right child nodes according to the node optimization criteria, such that to minimize the uncertainties of the class-conditional distributions $p(\mathbf{d}|c)$ and the class label $p(c)$. Only class-conditional distributions $p(\mathbf{d}|c)$ of the myocardium and the blood pool participate in the training. Each leaf node stores the discrete class label distribution $p(c)$ and the distance vectors $\mathbf{d}_c$.

arrived at this node. Randomness is injected via a small number of randomly selected features (m = 100) at each node.

Node Optimization. Each split node is assigned a binary test, which is defined as

$$h(\mathbf{v}) = \lfloor f_i(\mathbf{v}) < \tau \rfloor \tag{1}$$

where $f_i \in \{f_1, f_2, \ldots, f_n\}$ is the feature associated with the node, and $\lfloor \cdot \rfloor$ is the indicator function. A set of m features is randomly selected from the pool of features $f = (f_1, f_2, \ldots, f_n)$, $t = 10$ random thresholds τ are tested per feature to find the pair (f_i, τ) that maximizes the objective function defined below.

The splitting minimizes the average uncertainty in the parameter values over the child nodes:

$$\min(p_{left} U^{left} + p_{right} U^{right}) \tag{2}$$

Note, that p_{left} and p_{right} should model the probabilities that a voxel will be sent to the left or to the right child node during *testing*, and not training. For example, if p_{left} is very small and p_{right} is large, the node split function will put its emphasis on minimizing the U^{right} uncertainty at the right child node. This is done with the assumption that most of datapoints at testing will be sent to the *right* child node, making U^{right} more important. In practice, the probabilities p_{left} and p_{right} are estimated as a proportion of the *training* voxels sent to the left and to the right child nodes. However, in many cases when the training datapoints are sampled to have a uniformly distributed class label, these estimations are incorrect due to the fact that no such sampling is possible at the testing stage. Therefore, we sample the training dataset uniformly regardless to the class label c, and estimate $p_{left} = \frac{|S^{left}|}{|S|}$ and $p_{right} = \frac{|S^{right}|}{|S|}$, where $|S^{left}|$ and $|S^{right}|$ are the number of datapoints sent to the left and to the right child nodes, $|S|$ is the number of datapoints in the parent node.

The ideal splitting should maximize the confidence of the predictors in the leaf nodes. In this work, we are interested in the weighted class-conditional parameter distributions $p(\mathbf{d}_c|c)p(c)$ (more details in Sect. 2.2), thus optimization should be both for $p(\mathbf{d}_c|c)$ and $p(c)$. We therefore define the following uncertainty measure for $p(\mathbf{d}_c|c)$ for the child nodes $l = \{left, right\}$:

$$U^l(S^l) = \sum_c U(S^l_c) p(c|S^l), \tag{3}$$

where $U(S^l_c)$ is the class-specific uncertainty of $\mathbf{d}_c$, chosen to encode the sample variance of $\mathbf{d}_c$:

$$U(S^l_c) = \frac{1}{|S^l_c| - 1} \sum_{\mathbf{d} \in S^l_c} (\mathbf{d} - \frac{1}{|S^l_c|} \sum_{\mathbf{d}' \in S^l_c} \mathbf{d}')^2 \tag{4}$$

Combining (2) (3) and (4) yields the following objective function:

$$U_{\mathbf{d}}(S) = \sum_{l=\{left, right\}} p^l \left(\sum_c p(c|S^l) \cdot \frac{1}{|S^l_c| - 1} \sum_{\mathbf{d} \in S^l_c} (\mathbf{d} - \frac{1}{|S^l_c|} \sum_{\mathbf{d}' \in S^l_c} \mathbf{d}')^2 \right) \tag{5}$$

For the class label uncertainty, we choose the average entropy of the class label distributions over the child nodes. Minimizing the entropy is equivalent to maximizing information gain.

$$U_c(S) = -\left|S^{left}\right| \cdot \sum_c p\left(c|S^{left}\right) - \left|S^{right}\right| \cdot \sum_c p\left(c|S^{right}\right) \tag{6}$$

Every split node randomly selects (5) or (6) to optimize either for class label c or the continuous parameters $\mathbf{d}_c$.

2.2 Testing

Given a new unseen image I, all voxels of that image are passed through the trees of the forest. Each voxel traverses the tree until it reaches a leaf node l. The voxel then votes for the location of the plane $\mathbf{b} = (b_1, b_2, b_3)$ using $p(c)$ and distance vectors $\mathbf{d}$ from the leaf. The parametrization of the plane $\mathbf{b}$ is expressed via the stored distance vectors $\mathbf{d}$, as shown in Fig. 2:

$$\mathbf{b} = \mathbf{d}\left(\frac{\mathbf{v} \cdot \mathbf{d}}{|\mathbf{d}|^2} + 1\right) \tag{7}$$

where $\mathbf{v}$ is the voxel.

We are interested in the probability $p(\mathbf{b}|l(\mathbf{v}))$, which can be decomposed as follows:

$$
\begin{aligned}
p(\mathbf{b}|l(\mathbf{v})) &= \sum_c p(\mathbf{b}|c, l(\mathbf{v})) p(c|l(\mathbf{v})) \\
&= \sum_c p\left(\mathbf{b} = \mathbf{d}_c\left(\frac{\mathbf{v} \cdot \mathbf{d}_c}{|\mathbf{d}_c|^2} + 1\right)|c, l(\mathbf{v})\right) p(c|l(\mathbf{v}))
\end{aligned} \tag{8}
$$

The distribution $p(c|l(\mathbf{v}))$ is estimated as the proportion of voxels per class c at the leaf, while $p(\mathbf{b}|c, l(\mathbf{v}))$ is estimated by a sum of Dirac measures $\delta_{\mathbf{d}}$ as in [1]:

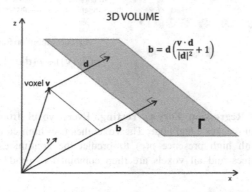

Fig. 2. Mapping from distance vectors $\mathbf{d}$ (distance from voxels to the plane) to the original plane parameters vector $\mathbf{b}$.

$$p(\mathbf{b}|l(\mathbf{v})) = \sum_c p(c|l(\mathbf{v})) \cdot \frac{1}{\left|S_c^{l(\mathbf{v})}\right|} \sum_{\mathbf{d} \in S_c^{l(\mathbf{v})}} \delta_{\mathbf{d}}\left(\mathbf{d}\left(\frac{\mathbf{v} \cdot \mathbf{d}}{|\mathbf{d}|^2} + 1\right)\right) \qquad (9)$$

Having separate class-conditional distributions $p(\mathbf{d}|c)$ allows for exclusion of distributions with the low confidence or low presence $p(c)$ from voting, Fig. 3. We choose the sample variance of $\mathbf{d}_c$ as the uncertainty measure and set a threshold K on it to control the maximum uncertainty of the participating distributions $p(\mathbf{d}_c)$. An additional threshold M on $p(c)$ is set to control the minimum presence of the class c at the leaf. The parameters K and M are found by cross-validation along with the maximum depth of the trees D. An example in Fig. 3 explains a possible voting scenario from a single voxel $\mathbf{v}$.

Once one or more class-conditional distributions $p(\mathbf{d}|c)$ are excluded from voting, the sum in (8) ceases to be a probability measure since it does not integrate to one. However, we are only interested in the maximum of $p(\mathbf{b}|l)$ in (10), which can be obtained without a normalization factor.

The votes from all voxels and all trees are collected to produce a single posterior probability distribution:

$$p(\mathbf{b}|I) \propto \sum_{\mathbf{v}} \sum_{t=1}^{T} \sum_{\hat{c}} p(\hat{c}|l(\mathbf{v})) \cdot \frac{1}{\left|S_{\hat{c}}^{l(\mathbf{v})}\right|} \sum_{\mathbf{d} \in S_{\hat{c}}^{l(\mathbf{v})}} \delta_{\mathbf{d}}\left(\mathbf{d}\left(\frac{\mathbf{v} \cdot \mathbf{d}}{|\mathbf{d}|^2} + 1\right)\right) \qquad (10)$$

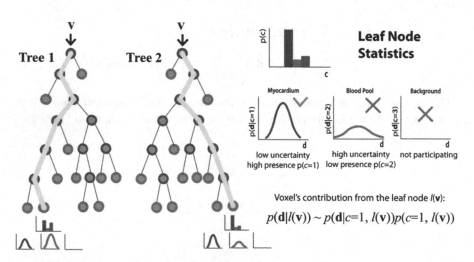

Fig. 3. Class-specific Regression Forest. Testing. Every voxel from the testing image traverses the tree until it reaches a leaf node. The voxel then uses high-confidence class-specific distributions $p(\mathbf{d}|c)$ with high presence $p(c)$ to predict the continuous output parameters. Predictions from all trees and all voxels are then combined to produce a single posterior probability.

where $\hat{c}$ is the class label whose corresponding distribution $p(\mathbf{d}|c, l)$ is included in the voting. The measure (10) is further smoothed with a Gaussian kernel G and the parameters of the plane are extracted as follows:

$$\mathbf{b}_{plane} = \mathbf{max_b}(p(\mathbf{b}|I) \circ G) \tag{11}$$

2.3   Features

Several classic low level local appearance features are adopted in this work, namely rectangle3D, Haar3D, and Difference3D features [8–10]. The Position3D feature is also employed to capture the absolute position of the voxels in the image.

3   Experimental Results

3.1   Dataset

25 end-diastolic 3D echocardiograms from healthy subjects were used in this study. A Philips iE33 ultrasound system was used to acquire the images. Volume dimensions are $224 \times 208 \times 208$ with an average of 0.88 mm^3 spatial resolution. The myocardium and the blood pool of all volumes, along with the 2C, 3C and 4C views were manually segmented/annotated by an expert.

3.2   Validation

Three class-specific regression forests and three classic regression forests were trained to detect 2C, 3C and 4C standard views from 3D Echocardiography. In each case, 20 volumes were chosen randomly for training and the remaining 5 volumes were used in testing.

To measure the similarity between two planes, two error metrics were utilized, namely, distance and angle.

The distance between two planes is defined as follows:

$$D = |\mathbf{b}_{automatic} - \mathbf{b}_{manual}| \tag{12}$$

where $\mathbf{b}_{automatic}$ and $\mathbf{b}_{manual}$ are the distances from the origin to the automatically detected plane and the manually annotated plane, Fig. 4.

The angle between two planes is measured as the angle between the normals to the planes:

$$\theta = \cos^{-1} \frac{\mathbf{n}_a \mathbf{n}_m}{|\mathbf{n}_a||\mathbf{n}_m|} \tag{13}$$

The performance of the class-specific regression forest summarized in Table 1. The results were obtained with the maximum tree depth D = 18, number of trees T = 12,

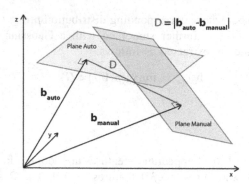

Fig. 4. Distance D is used to compare the performance of the classic regression forest with the performance of the class-specific regression forest.

Table 1. Distance in millimetre and angle in degrees using the traditional and the class-specific regression forests for the 2C, 3C and 4C planes.

		2 chamber	3 chamber	4 chamber
Distance	Traditional RF	14.0 ± 10.7	15.0 ± 8.7	13.8 ± 9.5
(mm)	Class-specific RF	5.5 ± 4.0	6.1 ± 4.0	5.2 ± 3.6
Angle	Traditional RF	6.4 ± 5.7	8.3 ± 6.3	6.2 ± 5.4
(degrees)	Class-specific RF	3.2 ± 2.2	3.4 ± 3.1	3.2 ± 2.0

width of the Gaussian kernel $\sigma^2 = 2\ mm$, m $= 100$ randomly chosen features where tested at each node during training. Only class-conditional distribution $p(d|c)$ with presence $p(c = myocardium) > 0.7$ for myocardium and $p(c = blood\_pool) > 0.8$ for blood pool were used in predictions.

The regression forests were implemented in C++. Testing one volume requires approximately 10 s using Intel Xeon 2.8 GHz computer with 12 cores and 48 GB RAM running Win7. With a parallel tree implementation, training required about 9 h and only needed to be done once.

4   Results

We report the mean $\pm$ standard deviation of the distance and angle in Table 1. The table shows comparisons between the classic regression forest and the class-specific regression forest on 2C, 3C and 4C standard views detection (Fig. 5). Examples of the detection results for 2C, 3C and 4C are shown in Fig. 3.

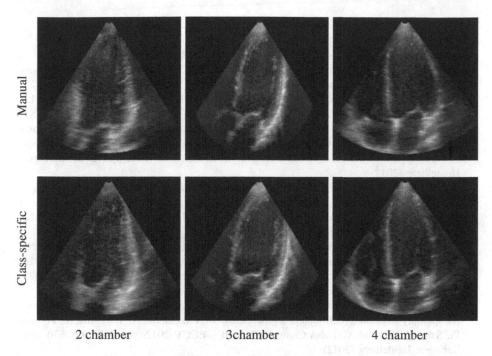

Fig. 5. Visual comparison between manual 2C, 3C and 4C planes (top row) and the automatically detected 2C, 3C and 4C planes (bottom row) using the class-specific regression forests.

5 Conclusions

We have presented an approach to the plane detection task using continuous parameterization and regression voting procedure. In the context of standard planes detection from 3D echocardiography, we proposed a class-specific regression forest, where additional structural information in the form of voxel class label was injected into the training step of the algorithm. Compared to the classic regression forest, a significant improvement has been observed. The boost in performance can be explained by the ability of the class-specific regression forest to localize the areas with meaningful to the problem information and ignore the extensive amount of irrelevant data from outside of the left and right ventricles. Future work includes incorporation of the right ventricle voxel classes into the algorithm and validation of the algorithm on a larger dataset.

Acknowledgement. This research was funded by the UK EPSRC on grant EP/G030693/1

References

1. Breiman, L.: Random forests. Mach. Learn. **45**, 5–32 (2001)
2. Criminisi, A., Shotton, J., Robinson, D., Konukoglu, E.: Regression forests for efficient anatomy detection and localization in CT studies. In: Menze, B., Langs, G., Tu, Z., Criminisi, A. (eds.) MICCAI 2010 Workshop MCV. LNCS, vol. 6533, pp. 106–117. Springer, Heidelberg (2010)
3. Konukoglu, E., Glocker, B., Zikic, D., Criminisi, A.: Neighbourhood approximation forests. In: Ayache, N., Delingette, H., Golland, P., Mori, K. (eds.) Medical Image Computing and Computer-Assisted Intervention. LNCS, vol. 7512, pp. 75–82. Springer, Heidelberg (2012)
4. Roberts, M.G., Cootes, T.F., Adams, J.E.: Automatic location of vertebrae on DXA images using random forest regression. In: Ayache, N., Delingette, H., Golland, P., Mori, K. (eds.) Medical Image Computing and Computer-Assisted Intervention. LNCS, vol. 7512, pp. 361–368. Springer, Heidelberg (2012)
5. Pauly, O., Glocker, B., Criminisi, A., Mateus, D., Moller, A.M., Nekolla, S., Navab, N.: Fast multiple organs detection and localization in whole-body MR dixon sequences. In: Fichtinger, G., Martel, A., Peters, T. (eds.) MICCAI 2011, Part III. LNCS, vol. 6893, pp. 239–247. Springer, Heidelberg (2011)
6. Glocker, B., Pauly, O., Konukoglu, E., Criminisi, A.: Joint classification-regression forests for spatially structured multi-object segmentation. In: Fitzgibbon, A., Lazebnik, S., Perona, P., Sato, Y., Schmid, C. (eds.) Computer Vision – ECCV 2012, vol. 7575, pp. 870–881. Springer, Heidelberg (2012)
7. Gall, J., Yao, A., Razavi, N., Van Gool, L., Lempitsky, V.: Hough forests for object detection, tracking, and action recognition. IEEE Trans. Pattern Anal. Mach. Intell. **33**, 2188–2202 (2011)
8. Geremia, E., Menze, B.H., Clatz, O., Konukoglu, E., Criminisi, A., Ayache, N.: Spatial decision forests for MS lesion segmentation in multi-channel MR images. In: Jiang, T., Navab, N., Pluim, J.P.W., Viergever, M.A. (eds.) MICCAI 2010, Part I, vol. 6361, pp. 111–118. Springer, Heidelberg (2010)
9. Yaqub, M., Javaid, K., Cooper, C., Noble, A.: Efficient volumetric segmentation using 3D fast-weighted random forests. In: MICCAI Workshop on Machine Learning in Medical Imaging, Toronto, Canada (2011)
10. Shotton, J., Johnson, M., Cipolla, R.: Semantic texton forests for image categorization and segmentation. In: Computer Vision and Pattern Recognition, pp. 1–8. Anchorage, AK, USA (2008)

Segmentation

Accurate Whole-Brain Segmentation for Alzheimer's Disease Combining an Adaptive Statistical Atlas and Multi-atlas

Zhennan Yan[1], Shaoting Zhang[1], Xiaofeng Liu[2], Dimitris N. Metaxas[1], Albert Montillo[2]([✉]), and The Australian Imaging Biomarkers and Lifestyle Flagship Study of Ageing[3]

[1] CBIM, Rutgers, The State University of New Jersey, Piscataway, NJ, USA
[2] GE Global Research, Niskayuna, NY, USA
montillo@ge.com
[3] Commonwealth Scientific and Industrial Research Organisation, Brisbane, Australia

Abstract. Accurate segmentation of whole brain MR images including the cortex, white matter and subcortical structures is challenging due to inter-subject variability and the complex geometry of brain anatomy. However a precise solution would enable accurate, objective measurement of structure volumes for disease quantification. Our contribution is three-fold. First we construct an adaptive statistical atlas that combines structure specific relaxation and spatially varying adaptivity. Second we integrate an isotropic pairwise class-specific MRF model of label connectivity. Together these permit precise control over adaptivity, allowing many structures to be segmented simultaneously with superior accuracy. Third, we develop a framework combining the improved adaptive statistical atlas with a multi-atlas method which achieves simultaneous accurate segmentation of the cortex, ventricles, and sub-cortical structures in severely diseased brains, a feat not attained in [18]. We test the proposed method on 46 brains including 28 diseased brain with Alzheimer's and 18 healthy brains. Our proposed method yields higher accuracy than state-of-the-art approaches on both healthy and diseased brains.

Keywords: Brain segmentation · Alzheimer's · Adaptive atlas · Multi-atlas · MRF

1 Introduction

The neurologic study and clinical diagnosis of many brain diseases, such as Alzheimer's Disease (AD) or hydrocephalus, often requires magnetic resonance

Data used in the preparation of this article was obtained from the Australian Imaging Biomarkers and Lifestyle flagship study of ageing (AIBL) funded by the Commonwealth Scientific and Industrial Research Organisation (CSIRO) which was made available at the ADNI database (www.loni.ucla.edu/ADNI). The AIBL researchers contributed data but did not participate in analysis or writing of this report. AIBL researchers are listed at www.aibl.csiro.au.

B. Menze et al. (Eds.): MCV 2013, LNCS 8331, pp. 65–73, 2014.
DOI: 10.1007/978-3-319-05530-5_7, © Springer International Publishing Switzerland 2014

(MR) imaging of the brain. Segmentation of distinct brain structures from MR images is a vital process for objective diagnosis, treatment planning, therapy monitoring and drug development. Manual labeling of brain structures in MR images by a human expert can require up to 1 week per subject and is operator dependent. For large data sets, manual segmentation of individual structures is not practical; however automating the segmentation is difficult due to image artifacts, noise, complex textures, complex shapes and partial volume effect. In recent decades, many approaches have been proposed to segment human organs or tissues in MR images or other modalities [11], for example classification based methods [6], deformable model based methods [10], and atlas-guided approaches [1, 7, 9, 12, 14, 16]. Among these approaches, atlas based methods are the most commonly used approaches for brain image segmentation. In medical image segmentation (e.g. [15]), an atlas is defined as a pair of an MR intensity scan (e.g. T1) and its corresponding manual segmentation. Given several atlases, there are two ways to segment a new target image. The first is to learn a single statistical atlas that models the spatial priors for individual structures. A single probabilistic atlas is fit in a Bayesian framework for voxel classification [1,14]. Single statistical atlas based methods are accurate when the target scan has similar anatomical characteristics as the atlas populations. The second approach is to register the set of atlases (multi-atlas) to the target image and then compute the final segmentation via a label fusion approach [7,9,12,16]. A multi-atlas method tends to be computationally expensive due to the required multiple non-linear registrations [2,17] and also has limited ability to handle diseased brains with anatomical characteristics that vary from the training atlases.

Recently, several adaptive statistical atlas-based expectation maximization (EM) algorithms were proposed to deal with the above limitation of atlas based methods. One by Shiee et al. [13] was applied to segment brains with ventriculomegaly. Another by Cardoso et al. [3] was applied to measure cortical thickness. In their work the brain is segmented into only 4–6 coarse structures: white matter (WM), gray matter (GM), ventricles, cerebrospinal fluid (CSF). However, the subcortical GM structures (e.g. hippocampus), which are critical in clinical diagnoses are not handled. In [18], we proposed an extended adaptive statistical atlas (EASA) using spatially varying adaptivity prior to segment many structures from whole brain MR scans, and use a strategy to combine the statistical atlas with multi-atlas to enhance the accuracy of segmenting diseased brains. This method can fail for some structures such as the cerebral cortex which is critical for disease detection (e.g. cortical thinning in AD). One reason is the use of a simplistic Markov Random Field (MRF) model that assumes every pair of voxel label arrangements has the same probability. This can lead to leaking, an unregulated, undesirable form of atlas adaptivity.

In this work, we segment the whole brain into 34 anatomical structures simultaneously and accurately by improving the adaptive atlas methods [13,18]. Our methodological contributions include: (1) structure specific relaxation along with the spatial adaptivity prior, (2) an isotropic pairwise class-specific MRF model, (3) a complete hybrid framework of our proposed method, denoted **EASA++**, with a multi-atlas approach which improves segmentation accuracy on diseased brains, especially for the cerebral cortex and ventricles. We evaluate our hybrid method *on 46 brains*. We *qualitatively* evaluate our results on all 46 brains including 19 with moderately enlarged ventricles, and *quantitatively* evaluate on 27 brains including 18 normal brains, and 9 AD brains with severely enlarged ventricles. Finally we compare our performance against state-of-the-art approaches such as FreeSurfer [5].

2   Methods

Background for the Extended Adaptive Single Statistical Atlas (EASA) and Weighted Majority Voting (WMV) multi-atlas methods. In [13] an EM-based adaptive single statistical atlas (ASA) brain segmentation method was proposed to address the common clinical situation in which the target brain to be segmented is poorly represented by the brains in the training set. This method assumes that the brain consists of K structures ($k = 1, \ldots, K$), the number of voxels in the T1 MR image is N ($i = 1, \ldots, N$), and that the intensity distribution of each structure follows a Gaussian distribution. The observed image is modeled by a K-component Gaussian Mixture Model (GMM) [14] with unknown parameters: the mixing coefficients π_{ik} and $\theta_k = (\mu_k, \sigma_k^2)$, where μ_k and σ_k^2 are the means and variances, respectively. The true label for voxel i is denoted as z_i (a $K \times 1$ binary-valued vector), while the prior probability that voxel i belongs to structure k is written as $p_i = (p_{i1}, \ldots, p_{iK})$, and its posterior probability as w_{ik}. Since brain structure labels are piecewise constant, a MRF prior on z_i's is incorporated to the complete model:

$$f(Z, X | \boldsymbol{\pi}, \boldsymbol{\theta}) = \frac{1}{Norm} \prod_{i=1}^{N} \prod_{k=1}^{K} (\pi_{ik} G(x_i; \theta_k))^{z_{ik}} \exp \left\{ -\beta \sum_{j \in N_i} \sum_{l=1, l \neq k}^{K} z_{ik} z_{jl} \right\}$$

where x_i is the intensity in target image at voxel i, $G(x_i; \theta_k)$ is the Gaussian model of structure k, $Norm$ is the MRF normalizer term and N_i is the 6-connected neighborhood of voxel i. The EM algorithm is used to solve the maximum a posteriori (MAP) estimation of parameters π_{ik} and θ_i. Assuming π_i follows a Dirichlet distribution and applying a Gaussian smooth filter on w_{ik}^t, they used $\pi_{ik}^{t+1} \approx (1 - \kappa) p_{ik} + \kappa (G * w_{ik}^t)$ to trade off spatial prior fidelity and the current EM estimate. The method in [13] is limited in that it can only parcellate 4 coarse anatomical classes (WM, GM, exterior CSF and ventricular CSF).

In [18] we extended ASA (denoted EASA) to parcellate many more (30+) structures throughout the brain. This was achieved through two steps. First we took the global invariant relaxation parameter $\kappa = 0.5$ and made it spatially *variant*. The spatially variant adaptivity map $\kappa(\mathbf{x}): \mathbb{R}^3 \mapsto \mathbb{R}$ depends on the coordinates of voxel $\mathbf{x} \in \mathbb{R}^3$. Second to segment diseased brains more accurately, we combined EASA with a multi-atlas label fusion approach called intensity weighted majority voting (WMV) [9]. WMV extends canonical majority voting label fusion by incorporating the intensity of the target subject to further guide the final label selection. This approach, which we denote simply as [18], applies the multi-atlas WMV to the target. This (1) generates a rough initial parcellation for subsequent EM-based EASA, and (2) enables the creation of ASA priors that are target subject specific since the multi-atlas WMV maps the training atlases to the target.

While [18] successfully extended ASA to segment 30+ structures the method's limitations include an inaccurate segmentation of structures, such as the cerebral-cortex and neighboring WM. There was also limited quantitative evaluation in [18]. In this paper we propose a new ASA approach, **EASA++**, and two new hybrid approaches, **Hybrid2** and **Hybrid3**, which address these methodological limitations and we perform a thorough quantitative evaluation of the impact of our new methods.

Our proposed EASA++ and hybrid approaches. Though the IBSR[1] atlas is extensively used in the brain segmentation literature, its manual labels contain errors including an over segmentation of cortical gray (exterior CSF voxels labeled as cortex). Consequently multi-atlas approaches, such as WMV, can fail to achieve good cortical GM parcellation because the propagated atlases consistently over segment the target's cortex. [18] does not improve cortical GM segmentation because all registered atlases are incorrect in the same way, causing low label entropy (high confidence) which would have otherwise triggered relaxation and subject-specific adaptivity. This motivates our first improvement to improve segmentation accuracy for cortex, external CSF, and WM, by making the spatially varying relaxation map $\kappa(\mathbf{x})$ dependent on the anatomical structure. This yields greater adaptivity for structures whose manually segmentation is problematic. *Formally, our new relaxation map is a function of location* $\mathbf{x}$ *and structure* k:

$$\kappa(\mathbf{x}, k) = \begin{cases} \alpha_1 \cdot \kappa(\mathbf{x}) & if(k = k_{ECSF}) \\ \alpha_2 \cdot \kappa(\mathbf{x}) & if(k \in \{k_{WM's}\}) \\ \kappa(\mathbf{x}) & otherwise \end{cases}$$

where the white matter structures, $k_{WM's}$ include left and right cerebral WM, $\alpha_1, \alpha_2 \in (0..1)$ are empirically determined structure specific relaxation coefficients. $\kappa(\mathbf{x})$ is computed via voxel label entropy: $H(\mathbf{x}) = \sum_{k=1}^{K} -r_k(\mathbf{x})\log(r_k(\mathbf{x}))$ where $r_k(\mathbf{x})$ is the rate that voxel $\mathbf{x}$ is labeled as k in training data. More relaxation is allowed at voxels with larger entropy and less where entropy is lower.

Studying the evolution of labels of [18], we observe that if the initial segmentation had miss-labeled a voxel as another similar-intensity class to the true label, then incorrect label can be propagated to neighboring voxels with similar intensity values. To suppress such error propagation, we replace the isotropic MRF of [18], with a pairwise class-specific MRF model:

$$f(Z, X | \boldsymbol{\pi}, \boldsymbol{\theta}) = \frac{1}{Norm} \prod_{i=1}^{N} \prod_{k=1}^{K} (\pi_{ik} G(x_i; \theta_k))^{z_{ik}} \exp\left\{-\sum_{j \in N_i} \sum_{l=1, l \neq k}^{K} \beta(l, k) z_{ik} z_{jl}\right\}$$

---

[1] http://www.cma.mgh.harvard.edu/ibsr/

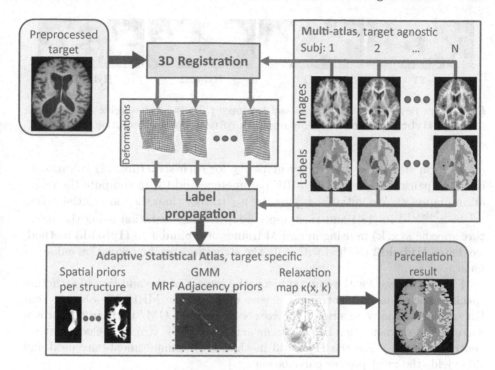

Fig. 1. Proposed **Hybrid3** algorithm first applies a multi-atlas to robustly initialize the segmentation and then applies an adaptive single statistical atlas for precise subject specific parcellation.

where $\beta(l, k)$ is the $K \times K$ MRF parameter matrix. These parameters are estimated in 3 steps. First for neighboring voxels throughout the whole atlas, we compute the pairwise class probability. Specifically we compute the probability that a voxel with label c2 appears next to the voxel with label c1 as $P_{pair}(c1, c2) = \frac{\# \text{ of pairs}(c1,c2)}{\# \text{ of voxels with label } c1}$ and average $P_{pair}(c1, c2)$ over all atlases. Finally we map $P_{pair}(c1, c2)$ to $\beta(c1, c2)$ values, where the larger the value of $P_{pair}(c1, c2)$ the smaller $\beta(c1, c2)$ should be to make the model have a larger probability of connecting classes. We model the relation as follows:

$$\beta(c1, c2) = \begin{cases} \frac{\gamma}{P_{pair}(c1,c2)} & \text{if } (P_{pair}(c1, c2) > \gamma) \\ 1 & \text{otherwise} \end{cases}$$

where $\gamma \in (0..1)$.

Having described **EASA++**, we combine it with multi-atlas method forming the new hybrid algorithm **Hybrid3**, which is illustrated in Fig. 1. After removing the skull using ROBEX [8], the preprocessed target (shown in the top left) is then non-linearly registered to each training scan using a diffeomorphic symmetric normalization [2]. The same transforms are used to propagate training subject label maps to the target. We combine these target specific label maps:

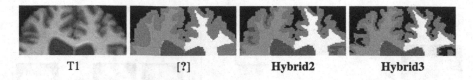

T1   [?]   **Hybrid2**   **Hybrid3**

Fig. 2. Our development of $\kappa(\mathbf{x}, \mathbf{k})$ and isotropic pairwise class-specific MRF for the proposed **Hybrid3** approach visibly improves cortical GM segmentation.

(1) to form statistical probability maps p_{ik} for each structure, (2) to estimate isotropic pairwise class-specific MRF parameters, and (3) to compute the relaxation map $\kappa(\mathbf{x})$. We initialize w_{ik}^0 by the p_{ik} (rather than the hard initialization $w_{ik}^0 = z_{ik}^{labelfus}$ in [18]) and then apply adaptive segmentation using the structure specific $\kappa(\mathbf{x}, \mathbf{k})$ in using in an EM framework. Similar to **Hybrid3** method, we define **Hybrid2** method with only the structure specific relaxation enhancement.

Figure 2 shows, for the same subject, the impact of the addition of structure specific relaxation and isotropic pairwise class-specific MRF. We observe that [18] mislabels many exterior CSF voxels as cortical GM. **Hybrid2** improves cortical GM segmentation but has some exterior to CSF voxels labeled as lateral ventricle (purple). For the **Hybrid3** method both enhancements are used and this yields the most precise parcellation.

3   Experiments

In this section, we evaluate the proposed **Hybrid3** method and compare it to state-of-the-art methods. We use two datasets. One is the IBSR data set which has 18 healthy subjects with T1 intensity volumes and medical expert delineated ground truth. Each brain volume has $256 \times 256 \times 128$ voxels, 1 mm in-axial plane resolution and 1.5 mm between-axial plane resolution. Each segmentation has 30+ labels including the left and right WM, GM, ventricles, and the subcortical GM structures (e.g. putamen, hippocampus, etc.). The other dataset consists of 28 Alzheimer's disease subjects randomly selected from the AIBL database[2]. Each brain volume has about $240 \times 256 \times 160$ voxels, 1 mm in-slice resolution and 1.2 mm between-slice resolution. The AIBL dataset consists of 9 subjects with severely enlarged lateral ventricles (denoted as Severe_AD) and 19 subjects with moderately enlarged lateral ventricles (denoted Moderate_AD). We manually labeled each subject volume in Severe_AD to provide ground truth for diseased brains.

In our first experiment we compared **EASA++**, **Hybrid3** to EASA and FreeSurfer on the IBSR dataset. From leave-one-out cross-validation tests, we observe overall best performance from the proposed **Hybrid3** method (see Fig. 3). The bar graph shows results from the first experiment and the second experiment (denoted as *_AD).

---

[2] Data was collected by the AIBL study group. AIBL study methodology has been reported previously ([4]).

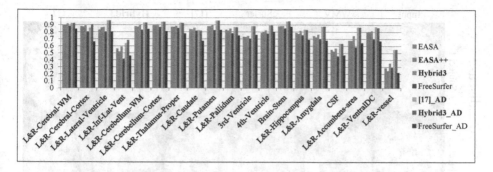

Fig. 3. Comparison of dice score per structure on 18 healthy subjects and 9 severe AD subjects. Proposed algorithm out performs benchmark methods such as FreeSurfer for most structures. 'L&R' stands for average result of structure in left and right spheres.

In our second experiment, we used the 18 healthy brains of IBSR as a training dataset and used the 28 subjects from the AIBL Alzheimer's disease dataset for testing. We evaluated and compared results of **Hybrid3** with FreeSurfer v5.1.0 and our implementation of WMV and [18]. For the **Hybrid3** approach we use empirically chosen parameters $\alpha_1 = 0.7$, $\alpha_2 = 0.9$, $\gamma = 0.001$. For quantitative evaluation, we compute average dice scores for 30+ structures in Severe_AD data set based on the ground truth. As shown in Fig. 3, the proposed approach yields better results than FreeSurfer in 27 out of 34 structures and **16 of these 27 are statistically significant differences by t-test,** ($p \leq 0.05$). These 16 structures include the Lateral Ventricles, which are known biomarkers for early detection of AD and can distinguish the stages of AD. FreeSurfer is **not** statistically significantly better for any structure. Comparing with [18], the proposed **Hybrid3** performs better for cerebral WM, cerebral cortex and ventricles. For general analysis, we recommend the **Hybrid3** approach as it works well for diseased **and** healthy appearing brains. Its computation time depends on the non-linear registrations performed to register atlases to target image and the number of training atlases. Once these registrations are performed (in parallel they take 30 min), the proposed algorithm only requires 7 minutes to segment one brain volume. For clinical practices where the subject is known to be similar in morphology to the set of training atlases, then our EASA or **EASA++** algorithm could be used alone (without the multi-atlas initialization step) in which case the entire segmentation requires just 7 minutes.

Qualitative results for two of Severe_AD subjects are shown in Fig. 4, while qualitative results for all 28 subjects are shown in the supplemental file. In Fig. 4, each row is for an axial slice of one subject in Severe_AD. The first column is the T1 input image; the second column is the result by WMV method; the third is FreeSurfer result; the fourth column comes from [18]; the fifth is the proposed **Hybrid3** result and the last column is ground truth (GT). The GT for each subject in Severe_AD is obtained by taking the WMV label fusion results as the starting point and manually re-labeling it. As shown by yellow circles in Fig. 4,

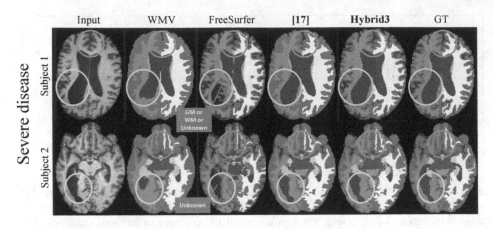

Fig. 4. Method comparison on AD patients. Proposed **Hybrid3** provides visibly improved parcellation (circled regions) throughout the brain

neither FreeSurfer, a statistical atlas method, nor WMV a multi-atlas method are able to reliably segment diseased ventricles. Blue circles indicate the areas where voxel based FreeSurfer under-segments the cortex, while yellow circles show where WMV and [18] over-segment the cortex. In our tests, *only **Hybrid3** is able to accurately segment the ventricles and cortex* of these diseased brains.

4   Conclusions and Future Work

We develop a new adaptive statistical atlas, **EASA++**, using structure specific relaxation priors, refined by a non-stationary relaxation map and isotropic pairwise class-specific MRF model. We propose a new hybrid approach **Hybrid3** that combines **EASA++** with the multi-atlas method. Our hybrid approach simultaneously segments 34 structures throughout the brain with state-of-the-art accuracy. We evaluate our method on normal brains and those with moderate and severe Alzheimer's. Qualitative and quantitative results demonstrate the superior performance of the proposed **Hybrid3** method to FreeSurfer for multiple structures including the cortex and ventricles. Since modern large datasets, such as ADNI and AIBL, have thousands of subjects, our fully automated proposed method is well suited for segmenting these images automatically across a wide range of disease severity. Future work entails improving accuracies for other small structures simultaneously and utilizing volumetry and thickness measures from our segmentations to quantify disease stage and help guide treatment.

References

1. Ashburner, J., Friston, K.: Unified segmentation. NeuroImage **26**, 839–851 (2005)
2. Avants, B., Epstein, C., Grossman, M., Gee, J.: Symmetric diffeomorphic image registration with cross-correlation: evaluating automated labeling of elderly and neurodegenerative brain. Med. Image Anal. **12**(1), 26–41 (2008)

3. Cardoso, M., Clarkson, M., Ridgway, G., Modat, M., Fox, N., Ourselin, S.: Load: a locally adaptive cortical segmentation algorithm. NeuroImage **56**(3), 1386–1397 (2011)

4. Ellis, K., et al.: The Australian imaging, biomarkers and lifestyle (AIBL) study of aging: methodology and baseline characteristics of 1112 individuals recruited for a longitudinal study of Alzheimer's disease. Int. Psychogeriatr. **21**(04), 672–687 (2009)

5. Fischl, B., Salat, D., Busa, E., Albert, M., et al.: Whole brain segmentation: automated labeling of neuroanatomical structures in the human brain. Neuron **33**(3), 341–355 (2002)

6. Gao, Y., Liao, S., Shen, D.: Prostate segmentation by sparse representation based classification. In: Ayache, N., Delingette, H., Golland, P., Mori, K. (eds.) MICCAI 2012, Part III. LNCS, vol. 7512, pp. 451–458. Springer, Heidelberg (2012)

7. Han, X., Hibbard, L., Oconnell, N., Willcut, V.: Automatic segmentation of parotids in head and neck CT images using multi-atlas fusion. In: MICCAI, pp. 297–304 (2010)

8. Iglesias, J., Liu, C., Thompson, P., Tu, Z.: Robust brain extraction across datasets and comparison with publicly available methods. TMI **30**(9), 1617–1634 (2011)

9. Liu, X., Montillo, A., Tan, E., Schenck, J.: iSTAPLE: improved label fusion for segmentation by combining STAPLE with image intensity. In: SPIE Medical Imaging (2013)

10. Mitchell, S., Bosch, J., Lelieveldt, B., van der Geest, R., Reiber, J., Sonka, M.: 3-d active appearance models: segmentation of cardiac MR and ultrasound images. TMI **21**(9), 1167–1178 (2002)

11. Pham, D.L., Xu, C., Prince, J.L.: Current methods in medical image segmentation. Annu. Rev. Biomed. Eng. **2**(1), 315–337 (2000)

12. Rousseau, F., Habas, P., Studholme, C.: A supervised patch-based approach for human brain labeling. TMI **30**(10), 1852–1862 (2011)

13. Shiee, N., Bazin, P.-L., Cuzzocreo, J.L., Blitz, A., Pham, D.L.: Segmentation of brain images using adaptive atlases with application to ventriculomegaly. In: Székely, G., Hahn, H.K. (eds.) IPMI 2011. LNCS, vol. 6801, pp. 1–12. Springer, Heidelberg (2011)

14. Van Leemput, K., Maes, F., Vandermeulen, D., Suetens, P.: Automated model-based tissue classification of MR images of the brain. TMI **18**(10), 897–908 (1999)

15. Wang, H., Suh, J.W., Das, S.R., Pluta, J., Altinay, M., Yushkevich, P.A.: Regression-based label fusion for multi-atlas segmentation. In: CVPR, pp. 1113–1120 (2011)

16. Warfield, S., Zou, K., Wells, W.: Simultaneous truth and performance level estimation (staple): an algorithm for the validation of image segmentation. TMI **23**(7), 903–921 (2004)

17. Wu, G., Kim, M., Wang, Q., Shen, D.: Hierarchical attribute-guided symmetric diffeomorphic registration for MR brain images. In: Ayache, N., Delingette, H., Golland, P., Mori, K. (eds.) MICCAI 2012, Part II. LNCS, vol. 7511, pp. 90–97. Springer, Heidelberg (2012)

18. Yan, Z., Zhang, S., Liu, X., Metaxas, D., Montillo, A., AIBL: accurate segmentation of brain images into 34 structures combining a non-stationary adaptive statistical atlas and a multi-atlas with applications to Alzheimer's disease. In: ISBI (2013)

Integrated Spatio-Temporal Segmentation of Longitudinal Brain Tumor Imaging Studies

Stefan Bauer[1](✉), Jean Tessier[2], Oliver Krieter[3], Lutz-P. Nolte[1],
and Mauricio Reyes[1]

[1] ISTB, University of Bern, Bern, Switzerland
[2] F. Hoffmann-La Roche Ltd., Basel, Switzerland
[3] Roche Diagnostics GmbH, Penzberg, Germany
stefan.bauer@istb.unibe.ch

Abstract. Consistent longitudinal segmentation of brain tumor images is a critical issue in treatment monitoring and in clinical trials. Fully automatic segmentation methods are a good candidate for reliably detecting changes of tumor volume over time. We propose an integrated 4D spatio-temporal brain tumor segmentation method, which combines supervised classification with conditional random field regularization in an energy minimization scheme. Promising results and improvements over classic 3D methods for monitoring the temporal volumetric evolution of necrotic, active and edema tumor compartments are demonstrated on a longitudinal dataset of glioma patient images from a multi-center clinical trial. Thanks to its speed and simplicity the approach is a good candidate for standard clinical use.

Keywords: Brain tumor · Glioma · Longitudinal studies · Segmentation · Volumetric analysis

1 Introduction

The segmentation of brain tumor images is an important clinical problem. It is necessary for patient monitoring and treatment planning, but it also has applications in clinical drug trials [9], where tumor response to therapy needs to be assessed. Many different automatic or semi-automatic segmentation algorithms have been proposed [5] and while their performance might be still debatable, it is well-accepted that manual segmentations are subject to high intra- and inter-rater variability [12]. This variability is even more influential when analysing longitudinal patient studies where tumor progression or regression should be monitored. In this case, it is more important to have an objective tumor segmentation, which can correctly identify changes over time, than having a very high accuracy at single time points. The RANO (response assessment in neuro-oncology) working group has pointed out, that in addition to the currently applied 2D manual diameter measurements for monitoring tumor growth, in the future it would be desirable to have reliable 3D measurements of volumetric

B. Menze et al. (Eds.): MCV 2013, LNCS 8331, pp. 74–83, 2014.
DOI: 10.1007/978-3-319-05530-5_8, © Springer International Publishing Switzerland 2014

tumor change [15]. Fully automatic segmentation algorithms are ideally suited for this scenario because they allow for an objective longitudinal assessment of tumor development. Furthermore they allow for an efficient handling of the large multi-modal datasets that are generated in longitudinal studies.

Despite the suitability of automatic methods for longitudinal studies, so far most algorithms for brain tumor segmentation have only been applied to images taken at single time points. Obviously, a standard segmentation algorithm for brain tumor images at single time points (e.g. [4,6,8,16]) could be applied for longitudinal studies, however this would not make use of the full temporal information, thus possibly decreasing robustness. There are only few methods, specifically designed for assessing temporal changes in brain tumor images, which mostly target slowly evolving low-grade gliomas. Konukoglu et al. [11] used a semi-automatic approach based on image registration for change detection. Pohl et al. [13] followed a similar idea, performing semi-automatic segmentation in combination with registration, after which they analyzed local intensity patterns to detect tumor growth. Angelini et al. [2] implemented a histogram mapping, which allowed them to compare intensity difference maps directly after affine registration.

Due to the irregular appearance and fast evolution of high-grade gliomas, registration methods are not well suited for this scenario. We chose a different approach for longitudinal brain tumor segmentation, which is based on supervised classification with integrated 4D spatio-temporal regularization for longitudinal brain tumor segmentation. It offers the possibility to segment tumor and healthy tissues including their subcompartments (necrotic, active, edema region and cerebrospinal fluid (CSF), gray matter (GM), white matter (WM) respectively).

2   Methods

The task is modeled as an energy minimization problem in a spatio-temporal conditional random field (CRF) formulation, where the random field contains cliques with both spatial and temporal links. The integration of spatial and temporal links was conceptually inspired by a work on video segmentation [14]. The energy consists of the sum of singleton potentials and pairwise potentials, which can be seen in the first and second term of Eq. (1), where i and j determine the voxel position in space and time. The optimization problem is solved to yield a segmentation result based on fast linear programming strategies [10].

$$E = \sum_i V(y_i, \mathbf{x}_i) + \sum_{ij} W(y_i, y_j, \mathbf{x}_i, \mathbf{x}_j) \tag{1}$$

The singleton potentials $V(y_i, \mathbf{x}_i)$ are computed according to Eq. (2), where y_i is the final label output, $\tilde{y}_i$ is the probability function learned from a discriminative classifier, $\mathbf{x}_i$ is the feature vector and δ is the Kronecker-δ function. For the classifier, a 40-dimensional feature vector $\mathbf{x}_i$ is used. It combines the normalized multi-modal intensities with first order textures (mean, variance,

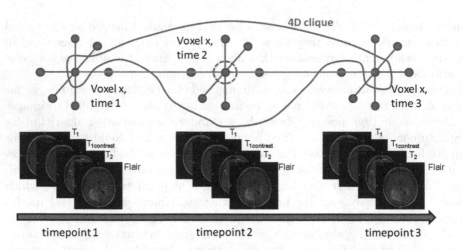

Fig. 1. The regularization is based on 4D spatio-temporal cliques for each voxel. The clique contains information from the local neighborhood of all image modalities at one time point, plus the previous and the subsequent time point.

skewness, kurtosis, energy, entropy) from local patches and statistics of gradient-based intensity differences in a local neighborhood.

$$V(y_i, \mathbf{x}_i) = p(\tilde{y}_i|\mathbf{x_i}) \cdot (1 - \delta(\tilde{y}_i, y_i)) \tag{2}$$

A decision forest classifier is employed because it can efficiently handle multi-label problems and provide posterior probabilities $p(\tilde{y}_i|\mathbf{x}_i)$ as an output [7]. This probabilistic output can be used as a weighting factor in Eq. (2), which allows us to control the degree of regularization depending on the confidence of the classification output.

The pairwise potentials $W(y_i, y_j, \mathbf{x}_i, \mathbf{x}_j)$ described in Eq. (3) account for the spatio-temporal regularization. In contrast to standard random field approaches, the cliques do not only model 3D spatial relationships, but 4D spatio-temporal relationships between image voxels, where each time frame is connected to the previous and the subsequent frame as illustrated in Fig. 1.

$$W(y_i, y_j, \mathbf{x}_i, \mathbf{x}_j) = w_s(i,j) \cdot (1 - \delta(y_i, y_j)) \cdot \exp\left(\frac{-\text{PCD}(\mathbf{x}_i, \mathbf{x}_j)}{2 \cdot \bar{x}}\right) \cdot D(y_i, y_j) \tag{3}$$

In Eq. (3), $w_s(i, j)$ is a weighting function that depends on the "spacing" in each dimension. This means the spatial resolution is taken into account, whereas for the temporal dimension a uniform spacing is chosen because depending on the treatment plan, changes in tumor volume do not necessarily depend on the imaging interval. Different labels of adjacent voxels are penalized by the term $(1 - \delta(y_i, y_j))$, whereas the degree of smoothing is regulated based on the local intensity variation, computed as $\exp\left(\frac{-\text{PCD}(\mathbf{x}_i, \mathbf{x}_j)}{2 \cdot \bar{x}}\right)$ with $\text{PCD}(\mathbf{x}_i, \mathbf{x}_j)$ being a pseudo-Chebyshev distance and $\bar{x}$ being the respective generalized mean intensity of the relevant modalities. The use of pseudo-Chebyshev distance is motivated by the fact that some modalities better describe certain tissues. In this case the $T_{1contrast}$ and Flair modalities are the most discriminative to distinguish the borders of individual tumor compartments and we make use of these two modalities only in the PCD term. Prior knowledge for penalizing different tissue adjacencies individually is taken into account by the $D(y_i, y_j)$ term in an empirical way. This allows us to stronger penalize adjacencies of tissues which are less likely to occur (e.g. necrotic and healthy tissue adjacencies).

3   Results

The method has been applied on an image dataset of 6 patients from a multi-center phase 1 clinical drug trial with a well-defined clinical image acquisition and drug administration protocol (part of the patients also had surgical resections). For each patient, there are 6 multi-modal MRI scans available at specific time points over a two-month period before and after drug ingestion (36 multi-modal images in total). This contains two baseline scans and four follow-up scans after treatment with anti-angiogenic therapies. Following the current clinical protocol, we operated only on the structural T_1, $T_{1contrast}$, T_2 and Flair MR images. The images of each patient were rigidly registered in order to ensure voxel-to-voxel correspondence and automatically skull-stripped in a pre-processing step. In our case, rigid registration was mandatory because we just aimed at aligning the brains to ensure general correspondence, internal tissue deformations caused by tumor growth or shrinkage were handled by the segmentation algorithm itself. Therefore they did not have to be considered by the registration method, otherwise the results of the volume measurements would be compromised. Additionally, bias-field correction, intensity normalization and denoising with an edge-preserving smoothing filter were performed.

We conducted two different experiments to evaluate the performance of the algorithm. First, we compared the proposed integrated 4D spatio-temporal segmentation to an enhanced version of the standard 3D segmentation from [3] (this was among the best performing methods at the MICCAI BraTS 2012 challenge and is basically the same as the approach presented here without considering temporal links in the regularization). The results were analyzed quantitatively by the overlap of the automatic segmentation result with a manually defined ground-truth using the Dice similarity coefficient and the mean surface distance. The Dice coefficient can range from 0 to 1 with 0 indicating no overlap and 1 indicating perfect overlap. The results are presented in Table 1. The average Dice coefficient increased when the spatio-temporal regularization was used. The increase was statistically significant for the active tumor region and partially also for the edema region (see Table 1). The added benefit of the 4D regularization is even more clear when considering the mean surface distance of the individual tumor compartments to the groundtruth. In almost all cases a clear significant improvement could be observed (see Table 1). The 3D segmentation tended to

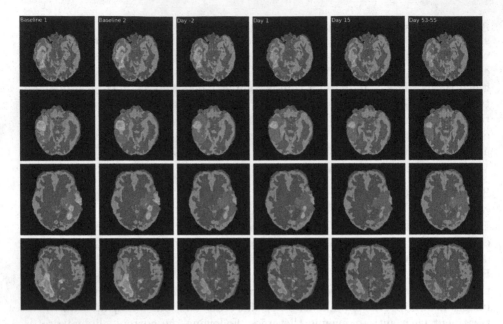

Fig. 2. Segmentation results for patient 2,3,5,6 from top to bottom (color code: red=CSF, green=GM, blue=WM, yellow=necrotic tumor, turquoise=active tumor, pink=edema). Each column shows one time point, starting from the first baseline scan, until the final scan 55 days after the first drug ingestion. (Results for patient 1 and 4 can be found in Figs. 4 and 5.)

produce strong outliers for the segmented volume at some time points. These could be effectively eliminated by the 4D regularization as can also be seen in Fig. 3, where the tumor volume evolution curves are more consistent with the clinical diagnosis for the 4D segmentation than the 3D segmentation. More details about some of the outliers generated by the 3D method in Fig. 3 are shown and further discussed in Figs. 4 and 5

Then, we evaluated the effect of different training datasets for the decision forest. Our standard training data were the training images of high-grade gliomas from the MICCAI 2012 BraTS challenge[1]. This is a dataset with a completely different image acquisition protocol than the one used for the longitudinal testing images. We wanted to see if the results improve when training is performed on a rough outline of the tumor on the first baseline image of each patient instead. As expected, it can be observed from Table 1 that the Dice coefficients are always higher when training is performed on the first baseline image of the same patient, but still the algorithm seems to generalize sufficiently well, so that even with training on the completely different BraTS dataset, acceptable results in terms of Dice overlap can be achieved. The rather low Dice coefficients for necrotic tissue can be explained by the fact that the necrotic region is often small

---

[1] http://www2.imm.dtu.dk/projects/BRATS2012/

Table 1. Average and standard deviation for overlap and surface distance of individual tumor compartments. Four different cases have been considered: training on BraTS with 3D segmentation, training on BraTS with 4D segmentation, training on the first baseline scan of the same patient with 3D segmentation, training on the first baseline scan of the same patient with 4D segmentation. Cases, where the 4D segmentation yielded a statistically significant improvement ($p < 0.05$) over the 3D segmentation have been marked with an asterisk

	3D BraTS	4D BraTS	3D baseline1	4D baseline1
Dice coefficient				
necrotic	0.18±0.22	0.18±0.21	0.45±0.35	0.45±0.35
active	0.54±0.2	0.58±0.18*	0.59±0.26	0.62±0.24*
edema	0.65±0.1	0.66±0.09	0.69±0.13	0.73±0.08*
Mean surface distance [mm]				
necrotic	15.6±14.9	10.5±9.4	5.5±6.7	2.1±2.1*
active	4.2±3.2	2.6±1.4***	2.9±3.8	1.8±2.9**
edema	4.7±3.2	3.5±1.9**	4.6±3.7	2.4±1.2***

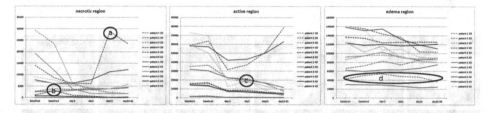

Fig. 3. Trend of the tumor volumes (in mm^3) for necrotic (left), active (center) and edema (right) compartments of all 6 patients. Results are shown with dashed lines for the pure 3D spatial segmentation and with solid lines for the proposed 4D spatio-temporal segmentation. The most prominent outliers of the 3D method are highlighted by black ellipses. Patient 4 showed progressive disease, which could be reliably identified from the computed active tumor region (purple line).

and the Dice coefficient is sensitive to the size of the region. Figure 2 illustrates the segmentation results on an axial slice of four patient images for all time points.

Finally, we compared the trend of the combined necrotic and active tumor volume, which was predicted by the algorithm, to the trend of the gross tumor volume, which had been manually outlined by an expert radiologist on the dynamic contrast enhanced (DCE) images of the same patient (these images were not used for the automatic segmentation method). The trend of the automatically segmented tumor volume is in general agreement with the tumor volumes manually defined on the DCE images, while the absolute values were still showing significant differences (see Fig. 6). The difference in absolute volume could be partially attributed to the fact that the resolution of our structural images was 4 times higher than the resolution of the DCE images, another explanation

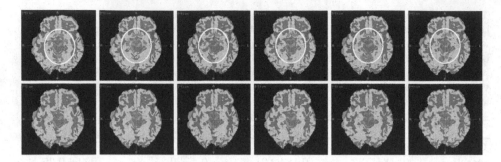

Fig. 4. Illustration of outlier (d) in Fig. 3 (edema region of patient 1). The upper row shows results of the 3D segmentation on one axial slice, the bottom row shows results of the 4D segmentation on the same axial slice. It can be seen that the pink edema region is changing location at every time point if the 3D segmentation method is used. This is not very likely and probably caused by acquisition artefacts. These artefacts are successfully suppressed by using the 4D segmentation method, leading to an edema volume which has a similar trend, but is generally lower than the volume given by the 3D segmentation method, as can be seen from Fig. 3.

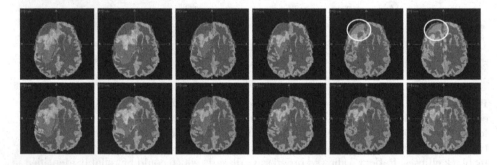

Fig. 5. Illustration of outlier (a) in Fig. 3 (necrotic region of patient 4). The upper row shows results of the 3D segmentation on one axial slice, the bottom row shows results of the 4D segmentation on the same axial slice. It can be seen that due to artefacts during image acquisition, a large fluid filled cavity is wrongly classified as being a necrotic tumor region (yellow) at the last two acquisition time points if the 3D segmentation method is used.

could be that structural images and functional DCE images contain different information.

Computation time on a multi-core CPU with 2.67 GHz was approximately 30 min for a 4-dimensional patient dataset, which translates to 5 min per single time point. This is in the range of the fastest state-of-the art algorithms for brain tumor segmentation.

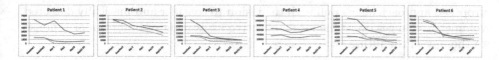

Fig. 6. Trend of the combined necrotic and active tumor volume, which was determined manually on the DCE images (blue line), and which was determined automatically from the four structural modalities, either with training on the BraTS data (red line) or with training on a rough manual tumor outline on the first baseline scan of each patient (green line). Results are shown in mm^3 for all 6 patients. Disease progression in patient 4 could be reliably identified.

4 Discussion and Conclusion

We presented a fully automatic method for integrated spatio-temporal segmentation of longitudinal brain tumor studies. The method is clinically oriented and can be easily used on the standard structural MRI modalities. To the best of our knowledge, this is the first automatic segmentation method, which is dedicated to longitudinal assessment of tumor progression or regression in high-grade glioma patients. It has many potential applications in radiology, oncology and clinical trials because it can eliminate the problem of non-objectiveness and user bias during evaluation and diagnosis.

We have demonstrated that a spatio-temporal segmentation has advantages over an independent treatment of all time points, exhibiting an increased robustness. This is specifically important for cases, where a large number of outliers occur at one time point due to either imaging artefacts or differences in image appearance. Such problems can be effectively handled by the temporal links of the cliques, yielding smoother and more informative curves for the volume trend. We acknowledge that this might lead to some bias by temporal smoothing, but that is outweighted by the improved robustness against outliers as shown qualitatively in Figs. 4, 5 and quantitatively by Dice scores and surface distances in Table 1. The presented method has the potential to allow for a more reliable diagnosis and assessment of tumor progression or regression. We have also shown that the trends of tumor volume evolution over time can be well captured by both intra- and inter-patient training, but obviously the results for intra-patient training are still more accurate.

Finally, we have been able to show that the automatic results for the longitudinal trend of the gross tumor volume, obtained from four structural imaging modalities only, correlated well with the longitudinal trend of the volumes, manually determined based on the DCE images. Additionally, the patient who clearly showed progressing disease could be reliably identified (see patient 4 in Fig. 3 center and in Fig. 6). The results obtained for the longitudinal tumor evolution were also in general agreement with clinical results reported by Ananthnarayan et al. [1] for patients exposed to treatment with an anti-angiogenic compound. Regarding the recommendations of the RANO group for assessing tumor evolution, the proposed approach aligns well with the vision to consider automatically detected volumetric changes over time for an effective assessment of brain tumor reponse to therapy in the future.

Acknowledgements. We would like to thank Roche for providing the image data including the manual measurements. This research was partially funded by the Swiss Institute for Computer Assisted Surgery (SICAS), the Swiss Cancer League and the Bernese Cancer League.

References

1. Ananthnarayan, S., Bahng, J., Roring, J., Nghiemphu, P., Lai, A., Cloughesy, T., Pope, W.B.: Time course of imaging changes of GBM during extended bevacizumab treatment. J. Neuro-Oncology **88**(3), 339–347 (2008)
2. Angelini, E., Delon, J., Bah, A.B., Capelle, L., Mandonnet, E.: Differential MRI analysis for quantification of low grade glioma growth. Med. Image Anal. **16**(1), 114–126 (2012)
3. Bauer, S., Fejes, T., Slotboom, J., Wiest, R., Nolte, L.P., Reyes, M.: Segmentation of brain tumor images based on integrated hierarchical classification and regularization. In: Menze, B., Jakab, A., Bauer, S., Reyes, M., Prastawa, M., Van Leemput, K. (eds.) Miccai Brats Workshop. Miccai Society, Nice (2012)
4. Bauer, S., Nolte, L.-P., Reyes, M.: Fully automatic segmentation of brain tumor images using support vector machine classification in combination with hierarchical conditional random field regularization. In: Fichtinger, G., Martel, A., Peters, T. (eds.) MICCAI 2011, Part III. LNCS, vol. 6893, pp. 354–361. Springer, Heidelberg (2011)
5. Bauer, S., Wiest, R., Nolte, L.P., Reyes, M.: A survey of MRI-based medical image analysis for brain tumor studies. Phys. Med. Biol. **58**(13), R97–R129 (2013)
6. Corso, J.J., Sharon, E., Dube, S., El-Saden, S., Sinha, U., Yuille, A.: Efficient multilevel brain tumor segmentation with integrated bayesian model classification. IEEE Trans. Med. Imaging **27**(5), 629–640 (2008)
7. Criminisi, A., Shotton, J., Konukoglu, E.: Decision forests for classification, regression, density estimation. manifold learning and semi-supervised learning. Tech. rep., Microsoft Research (2011)
8. Gooya, A., Pohl, K.M., Bilello, M., Cirillo, L., Biros, G., Melhem, E.R., Davatzikos, C.: GLISTR: glioma image segmentation and registration. IEEE Trans. Med. Imaging **31**(10), 1941–1954 (2012)
9. Henson, J.W., Ulmer, S., Harris, G.J.: Brain tumor imaging in clinical trials. AJNR. Am. J. Neuroradiol. **29**(3), 419–424 (2008)
10. Komodakis, N., Tziritas, G., Paragios, N.: Performance vs computational efficiency for optimizing single and dynamic MRFs: setting the state of the art with primal-dual strategies. Comput. Vis. Image Underst. **112**(1), 14–29 (2008)
11. Konukoglu, E., Wells, W., Novellas, S., Ayache, N., Kikinis, R., Black, P., Pohl, K.: Monitoring slowly evolving tumors. In: IEEE ISBI 2008, pp. 812–815. IEEE (2008)
12. Mazzara, G.P., Velthuizen, R.P., Pearlman, J.L., Greenberg, H.M., Wagner, H.: Brain tumor target volume determination for radiation treatment planning through automated MRI segmentation. Int. J. Radiat. Oncol. Biol. Phys. **59**(1), 300–312 (2004)

13. Pohl, K.M., Konukoglu, E., Novellas, S., Ayache, N., Fedorov, A., Talos, I.F., Golby, A., Wells, W.M., Kikinis, R., Black, P.M.: A new metric for detecting change in slowly evolving brain tumors: validation in meningioma patients. Neurosurgery 68(1 Suppl Operative), 225–233 (2011)
14. Wang, Y., Loe, K.F., Wu, J.K.: A dynamic conditional random field model for foreground and shadow segmentation. IEEE Trans. Pattern Anal. Mach. Intell. 28(2), 279–289 (2006)
15. Wen, P.Y., Macdonald, D.R., Reardon, D.A., Cloughesy, T.F., Sorensen, A.G., Galanis, E., Degroot, J., Wick, W., Gilbert, M.R., Lassman, A.B., Tsien, C., Mikkelsen, T., Wong, E.T., Chamberlain, M.C., Stupp, R., Lamborn, K.R., Vogelbaum, M.A., van den Bent, M.J., Chang, S.M.: Updated response assessment criteria for high-grade gliomas: response assessment in neuro-oncology working group. J. Clin. Oncol.: Official J. Am. Soc. Clin. Oncol. 28(11), 1963–1972 (2010)
16. Zikic, D., et al.: Decision forests for tissue-specific segmentation of high-grade gliomas in multi-channel MR. In: Ayache, N., Delingette, H., Golland, P., Mori, K. (eds.) MICCAI 2012, Part III. LNCS, vol. 7512, pp. 369–376. Springer, Heidelberg (2012)

Robust Mixture-Parameter Estimation for Unsupervised Segmentation of Brain MR Images

Alfiia Galimzianova[✉], Žiga Špiclin, Boštjan Likar, and Franjo Pernuš

Faculty of Electrical Engineering, University of Ljubljana, Ljubljana, Slovenia
{alfiia.galimzianova,ziga.spiclin,
bostjan.likar,franjo.pernus}@fe.uni-lj.si

Abstract. Methods for automated segmentation of brain MR images are routinely used in large-scale neurological studies. Automated segmentation is usually performed by unsupervised methods, since these can be used even if different MR sequences or different pathologies are studied. The unsupervised methods model intensity distribution of major brain structures using mixture models, the parameters of which need to be robustly estimated from MR data and in presence of outliers. In this paper, we propose a robust mixture-parameter estimation that detects outliers as samples with low significance level of the corresponding mixture component and iteratively re-estimates the fraction of outliers. Results on synthetic and real brain image datasets demonstrate superior robustness of the proposed method as compared to the popular FAST-TLE method over a broad range of trimming fraction values. The latter is important for segmenting brain structures with pathology, the extent of which is hard to predict in large-scale imaging studies.

Keywords: Mixture model · Robust estimation · Trimmed likelihood estimation · Expectation-maximization · Magnetic resonance imaging (MRI) · Brain · Segmentation · Outlier detection

1 Introduction

Diagnosis and follow-up of many neurological disorders are based on analysis of a set of magnetic resonance (MR) images of the brain. The analysis of brain MR images usually involves extraction of qualitative and quantitative information about brain tissues, fluids and pathologies by means of their manual detection and delineation, or segmentation. Manual segmentation of MR images, however, is both challenging (3D, multi-sequence MRI) and a time-consuming task, and is also subjected to considerable inter- and intra-rater variability. Therefore, in large-scale clinical studies automated methods are required to segment brain MR images. The segmentations obtained by the automated methods need to be robust and reproducible and should achieve accuracy level comparable to manual expert segmentations.

Methods for automated segmentation are usually classified as unsupervised and supervised. The latter incorporate *a priori* knowledge from manual expert

B. Menze et al. (Eds.): MCV 2013, LNCS 8331, pp. 84–94, 2014.
DOI: 10.1007/978-3-319-05530-5_9, © Springer International Publishing Switzerland 2014

segmentations of a large cohort of patients, but in brain MR image segmentation they have been applied with limited success mainly due to large variability in the position and appearance of different brain pathologies and due to large variability between MR acquisitions in multicenter clinical studies. Conversely, the unsupervised methods, which use only the patient's MR data to perform segmentation, are less dependent on the type of pathology and thus more attractive for large-scale multicenter studies.

Motivated by good contrast between different structures in brain MR images, the unsupervised methods usually employ an intensity model of major brain structures. The intensity model is represented by a mixture of distributions that correspond to the intensities of major brain tissues, such as white matter (WM), gray matter (GM), and cerebrospinal fluid (CSF). Most frequently, the intensity models are mixtures of Gaussian distributions [1, 2], but other distributions such as Student's-t [3], and Rician [4] were also used. Estimation of the intensity-model parameters is usually performed by the maximum-likelihood expectation-maximization (ML-EM) method [5]. However, the ML-EM method is known to be sensitive to unmodeled samples or outliers in the data. In modeling the MR intensities of WM, GM and CSF, the outliers appear on the borders between the modeled structures, known as the partial volume effect, and as a result of pathologies not captured by the intensity model. Hence, the method of outlier detection crucially defines the sensitivity, or robustness, of the unsupervised methods.

Several robust alternatives to the ML-EM method for brain MR image segmentation have been proposed that incorporate statistical proximity-based outlier detection [6]. Leemput et al. [1] modified the ML-EM method for Gaussian mixture models (GMM) by re-weighting the intensity samples based on typicality of a sample with respect to (w.r.t.) the component distribution. Neykov et al. [7] proposed a trimmed likelihood estimator (TLE), in which a fraction H of samples are considered as outliers and are removed in each iteration from the estimation of the mixture-components parameters. An efficient variant of the method, the so-called FAST-TLE selects the outlier samples from among the samples with the smallest log-likelihood. Several authors applied the FAST-TLE method [7] and proposed different proximity measures to capture the outliers [2, 8, 9]. The method by Leemput et al. [1] does not necessarily increase the likelihood of the intensity model in each iteration, while the FAST-TLE has guaranteed convergence in terms of model likelihood, but requires a careful selection of the trimming fraction H.

Trimming fraction H should correspond to the actual outlier fraction. As such, using fixed value of H can significantly affect the performance of automated segmentation, thus it should be either assessed during or before the likelihood maximization process. The techniques proposed to assess the optimal value of H [7, 10] require that the likelihood maximization is run for several values of the trimming fraction. These techniques drastically increase the computational complexity of the likelihood maximization and as such are not suitable for large-scale brain MR image processing. Garcia-Lorenzo et al. [2] set trimming fractions higher than the actual outlier fraction and obtained relatively stable mixture-parameter estimations. However, when H is much higher than the actual outlier fraction the TL estimation is no longer accurate and the mixture-parameter estimation becomes biased.

In this paper, we propose a new method for robust mixture-parameter estimation that iteratively re-estimates the trimming fraction H and is more stable to the given initial value. Unlike the FAST-TLE method [7], which detects outliers as samples with low log-likelihoods of the mixture distribution, the proposed method detects outliers as samples with low significance levels w.r.t. the corresponding mixture component. The trimming fraction H is adaptively increased at each iteration so that the likelihood increases at each iteration. We demonstrate that the proposed modifications result in a more robust mixture-parameter estimation than the FAST-TLE for a broad range of values of the trimming fraction. This is especially important for the task of segmentation of brain tissues in the presence of outliers such as pathologies, the extent of which is very hard to predict in large-scale multicenter imaging studies.

2 Methods

Let $\{x_1, \ldots, x_N\}$ represent vector-valued intensity samples of multi-sequence MR images sampled from corresponding locations in the space domain Γ; $card(\Gamma) = N$. Consider x_j are samples of i.i.d. random vectors, drawn from a mixture of K distributions $p_k(x|\theta_k)$, with component priors $\pi_k > 0$, $k = 1, K$, defined by

$$\psi(x|\Theta) = \sum_{k=1}^{K} \pi_k p_k(x|\theta_k),$$ (1)

where $\Theta = \{\pi_1, \ldots, \pi_K, \theta_1, \ldots \theta_K\}$ is a vector of unknown mixture parameters, and the component priors always sum to one ($\sum_{k=1}^{k} \pi_k = 1$). Density function $\psi(x|\Theta)$ represents the intensity model of normal-appearing major brain structures. The EM method [5] is used to estimate the parameters of intensity model in (1) so that the log-likelihood function of the intensity model is maximized

$$l(\Theta) = \sum_{j=1}^{N} \log \psi(x_j|\Theta).$$ (2)

2.1 Mixture-Parameter Estimation by FAST-TLE

When samples x_j are contaminated by outliers, the parameter estimation can be formulated as maximization of the trimmed likelihood (TL) function defined as

$$TL(\Theta|v, H) = \sum_{j=1}^{N-\lfloor HN \rfloor} \log(\psi(x_{v_j}|\Theta)),$$ (3)

where H is the trimming fraction, $\lfloor \cdot \rfloor$ is a floor function, and $v = \{v_1, \ldots, v_N\}$ is a permutation of indices $j = \{1, \ldots, N\}$ corresponding to the following ordering of samples

$$\log(\psi(x_{v_1}|\Theta)) \geq \log(\psi(x_{v_2}|\Theta)) \geq \cdots \geq \log(\psi(x_{v_N}|\Theta)).$$ (4)

Hence, in FAST-TLE [7] the $\lfloor HN \rfloor$ samples with smallest log-likelihoods are removed in each iteration from the trimmed likelihood maximization.

The maximization of (3) is performed by EM using the remaining samples to yield new mixture-parameter estimates, then the set of trimmed samples are reset according to the current intensity model. In this way, the method improves at each iteration the previous estimate of the trimmed likelihood (3) and leads to a suboptimal approximation of the maximum of true TL function.

FAST-TLE can produce robust mixture-parameter estimates only when the trimming fraction H is set slightly higher than the true outlier fraction [2, 10]. If the trimming fraction H is set too high, then even the most representative samples corresponding to mixture components with small prior π_k will have low log-likelihoods and will thus be trimmed from the likelihood estimation (Fig. 1a).

2.2   Mixture-Parameter Estimation by Significance-Level Trimming

To address the mixture-parameter estimation for low component priors and the sensitivity of FAST-TLE to setting of the trimming fraction we propose two modifications to the original FAST-TLE. First, we alter the ordering rule in (4) so that instead of the joint log-likelihood of current mixture-parameter estimates the ordering considers component-wise significance levels. As shown in Fig. 1b the significance-level ordering preserves mixture components with low priors.

Outliers of the mixture model are usually defined as samples that correspond to low significance levels of the mixture component, to which they most likely belong to according to some classification rule. For instance, outliers from GMM are usually found by a threshold on Mahalanobis distance, which can be transformed to a significance level using chi-square law. Therefore, significance levels of corresponding mixture component are used for the ordering rule as

$$\int_{\Omega\left(x_{v_1}\right)} p_{z_{v_1}}\left(\omega|\Theta_{z_{v_1}}\right)d\omega \geq \cdots \geq \int_{\Omega\left(x_{v_N}\right)} p_{z_{v_N}}\left(\omega|\theta_{z_{v_N}}\right)d\omega \tag{5}$$

where $\Omega(x_j) = \{\omega \in \Omega : p_{z_j}\left(\omega|\theta_{z_j}\right) \leq p_{z_j}\left(x_j|\theta_{z_j}\right)\}$ with Ω being a sample space, and $z_j \in \{1, ..., K\}$ is a labeling of the samples according to the chosen classifier.

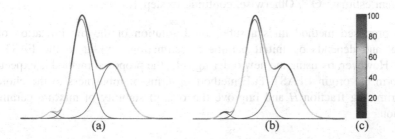

Fig. 1. Color coded order of the samples obtained from theoretical distribution of a three-component Gaussian mixture (a) according to the log-likelihood, and (b) according to significance levels of corresponding mixture components. The color coding follows (c) the scale of corresponding quantiles. Observe that the ordering according to significance levels treats samples of all components of the mixture equally regardless of value of their prior (Color figure online).

Second, as the modified ordering and trimming of samples in general does not guarantee the convergence to maximum TL mixture-parameter estimate, we adaptively increase the trimming fraction H at each iteration so that the trimmed likelihood also increases at each iteration. In the following, we describe a mixture-parameter estimation method based on the ordering rule in (5). Given the initial estimation of the mixture model parameters in (1), i.e. $\Theta^{(0)} = \{\pi_1^{(0)}, \ldots \pi_K^{(0)}, \theta_1^{(0)}, \ldots, \theta_K^{(0)}\}$ and the initial trimming fraction $h^{(0)} = H$, the iterations $i \geq 1$ consist of the following steps:

1. Based on the previous mixture-parameter estimates $\Theta^{(i-1)}$ and the corresponding labeling of the brain structures, permute the indices $\tilde{v} = \{\tilde{v}_1, \ldots, \tilde{v}_N\}$ of samples x_j according to (5). Obtain new mixture-parameter estimates by EM of the trimmed likelihood function with trimming fraction $h^{(i-1)}$

$$\Theta^{(i)} = arg \max_{\theta} TL\left(\Theta | \tilde{v}, h^{(i-1)}\right).$$

2. Based on the permutation $\tilde{v}$ found in the previous step, set the new value of trimming fraction $h^{(i)}$ by increasing $h^{(i-1)}$ until TL function in (3) is increased

$$h^{(i)} : TL\left(\Theta^{(i)} | \tilde{v}, h^{(i)}\right) \geq TL\left(\Theta^{(i)} | \tilde{v}, h^{(i-1)}\right)$$

To prevent $h^{(i)}$ from increasing to an unreasonable value, we set an upper bound on the trimming fraction based on initial trimming fraction H. Since for any permutation $\bar{v}$ of the indices $j = \{1, \ldots, N\}$

$$TL(\Theta | \bar{v}, h) \leq TL(\Theta | v, h)$$

where v is a permutation defined by the ordering rule in (4), we find the value of the trimming fraction that obeys $TL(\Theta) \leq TL\left(\Theta^{(i)} | \tilde{v}, H\right)$.

3. If $\left(TL\left(\Theta^{(i)} | \tilde{v}, h^{(i)}\right) - TL\left(\Theta^{(i-1)} | \tilde{v}, h^{(i-1)}\right)\right) / TL\left(\Theta^{(i-1)} | \tilde{v}, h^{(i-1)}\right) < \delta$, with δ being a predefined threshold, or $h^{(i-1)} - h^{(i)} = 0$, then terminate and return the current estimate $\Theta^{(i)}$. Otherwise, continue to step 1.

The proposed method finds a suboptimal solution of the maximization of TL function, and depends on initial parameter estimation, similar to the FAST-TLE method. However, by using the new ordering rule, the proposed method is expected to outperform the original FAST-TLE method in terms of robustness to the choice of initial trimming fraction H and improve the overall stability of mixture-parameters estimation.

3 Experiments and Results

In this section, we evaluate the performance of the proposed method and compare it to the FAST-TLE method [7]. Numerical simulations are performed in Sect. 3.1 to demonstrate the performance and convergence of the proposed method for different values of the trimming fraction H. In Sect. 3.2 segmentation of brain structures is performed on synthetic and real MR image datasets to demonstrate the application the proposed method.

3.1 Numerical Simulations

Performance and convergence properties of the proposed and the FAST-TLE methods for different values of the trimming fraction H were verified by generating inlier and outlier data points from two known overlapping distributions. There were 10^4 inliers sampled from the 3-component GMM with the following parameters

$$\pi_1 = 0.1, \pi_2 = 0.5, \pi_3 = 0.4$$

$$\mu_1 = (0\ 3)^T, \mu_2 = (3\ 0)^T, \mu_3 = (-3\ 0)^T$$

$$\Sigma_1 = \begin{pmatrix} 2 & 0.5 \\ 0.5 & 0.5 \end{pmatrix}, \Sigma_2 = \begin{pmatrix} 0.1 & 0 \\ 0 & 0.1 \end{pmatrix}, \Sigma_3 = \begin{pmatrix} 2 & -0.5 \\ -0.5 & 0.5 \end{pmatrix},$$

and $2 \cdot 10^3$ outliers ($H_{true} \approx 0.17$) generated from a uniform distribution in the range -10 to 10 in each dimension. The sample-generation model is similar to the one considered in [7], except that we used unequal component priors.

We tested the original FAST-TLE and the proposed methods, the parameters of both were initialized using the k-means method with 3 components. Trimming fraction was varied in the range $H \in \{0.15, 0.20, \ldots 0.4\}$ and the final mixture-parameter estimates were investigated. As can be seen from Fig. 2, when the values of trimming fraction were close to the true outlier fraction, the estimates produced by both methods were close to the true mixture model parameters. For higher values of the trimming

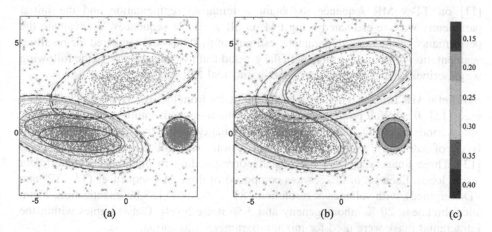

Fig. 2. Estimates of the Gaussian mixture model by (a) FAST-TLE method and (b) proposed method using (c) different trimming fraction values. The ellipses overlaid on the data points represent 99 % confidence intervals of the mixture components. The true model is represented by dashed ellipses. The inliers are shown as dots and outliers as crosses, respectively (Color figure online).

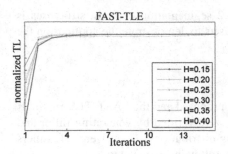
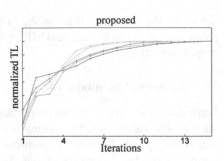

Fig. 3. Convergence of the trimmed likelihood (TL) function using original FAST-TLE and the proposed method on different values of trimming fraction H (Color figure online).

fraction (e.g. $H \geq 0.30$) the component with smallest prior was trimmed by the original FAST-TLE method, while the proposed method successfully captured this component even for higher values of the trimming fraction. The corresponding behavior of the TL function (3) over the first 15 iterations is shown in Fig. 3. Even though the proposed method has a slightly slower convergence compared to FAST-TLE, the TL increases with the iterations, indicating convergence.

3.2 Brain MR Images

In this section, we apply the proposed method and the FAST-TLE method to segment brain structures in MR images. GMM was used as intensity model of the major brain structures (WM, GM, CSF). Outliers of the intensity model mainly corresponded to image artifacts, such as partial volume effect, noise and pathology, such as brain lesions. To initialize the mixture parameters, we applied Otsu's thresholding method [11] on T1-w MR sequence to obtain a tentative segmentation and the initial parameters were re-estimated using EM on all available sequences. To evaluate the performance of the mixture-parameter estimation methods, we compared the resulting segmentation of brain structures with the ground truth segmentations. In the following we describe the experiments on synthetic and real MR images.

Synthetic MR Images. Publicly available datasets from the BrainWeb simulator were used [12]. BrainWeb provides digital brain phantoms with multi-sequence MR images, various intensity inhomogeneities and image noise levels, and with different levels of pathology, expressed as different lesion loads (mild, moderate, and severe) [12]. Three image sets were used, each corresponding to phantoms with different lesion loads. Each set of images was composed of three MR sequences (T1-, T2- and PD-weighted), with volumes of resolution $181 \times 217 \times 181$, 8 bit quantization, 1 mm slice thickness, 20 % inhomogeneity and 3 % noise levels. Only samples within the intracranial mask were used for mixture-parameter estimation.

First, we qualitatively investigated the behavior of the estimation methods under different values of the trimming fraction H. Intensity samples that were detected as outliers and excluded from TL function for trimming fractions of 0.05 and 0.20 are shown in Fig. 4b and c, respectively. While for small trimming fractions the maps of

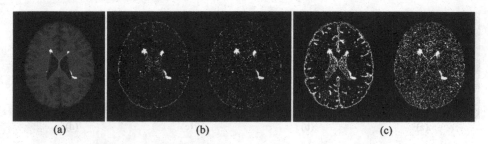

(a)   (b)   (c)

Fig. 4. BrainWeb phantom with moderate lesion (slice 96): (a) ground truth segmentation with lesions encoded in white color (b) and (c) show outlier samples as detected by FAST-TLE and the proposed methods, on the *left* and *right*, respectively; (b) trimming fraction $H = 0.05$ and (c) trimming fraction $H = 0.20$. Note in (c) the false outliers from CSF detected by the FAST-TLE, which is overcome by the proposed method.

outliers are relatively similar and primarily include samples that belong to lesions and noise, the maps corresponding to higher values differ considerably. The original FAST-TLE detected a high number of samples corresponding to CSF as outliers, which had the smallest prior in this case (Fig. 4c, *left*). Conversely, the proposed method correctly detected the lesion voxels and noise as outliers (Fig. 4c, *right*).

Second, the performance of the two methods was quantitatively evaluated by comparing the resulting segmentations of CSF, GM and WM to the corresponding ground truth segmentations. An unsupervised Bayesian classifier was used to obtain the segmentations, while Dice similarity coefficient (DSC) [13] was used as an evaluation measure. The DSC values for CSF, GM and WM, averaged over the phantoms with different lesion loads, are shown in Fig. 5. The variation of DSC for different trimming fractions indicates more stable performance of the proposed method compared to the FAST-TLE method.

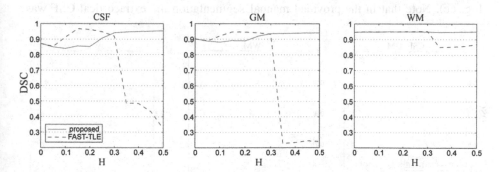

Fig. 5. Performance of the Bayesian-classification based segmentation using mixture-parameter estimates obtained by the FAST-TLE (*in dashed blue*) and the proposed method (*in solid red*) on BrainWeb phantoms. *From left to right*: Dice similarity coefficients (DSC) for cerebrospinal fluid (CSF), gray matter (GM) and white matter (WM), averaged over the phantoms with different lesion loads, over different values of trimming fraction H (Color figure online).

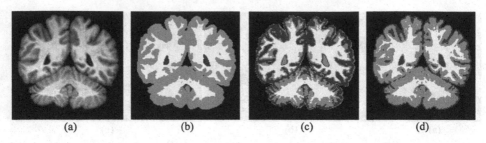

(a)   (b)   (c)   (d)

Fig. 6. Segmentations of the real brain MR image (IBSR07, slice 40). (a) T1-w MR image (b) ground truth segmentation with WM, GM and CSF encoded from brightest to darkest label (c) segmentation by FAST-TLE with trimming fraction $H = 0.5$ (d) segmentation by the proposed method with trimming fraction $H = 0.5$.

Real Brain MR Images. Normal brain MR images of 18 healthy subjects from publicly available Internet Brain Segmentation Repository (IBSR) provided by the Center for Morphometric Analysis at Massachusetts General Hospital [14] were used for testing the performance of mixture-parameter estimation. The performance was measured indirectly by comparing the obtained segmentations with the manual ground truth.

For each patient, the T1-weighted MR image with resolution of $256 \times 256 \times 128$, 1.5 mm slice thickness was provided. The mixture-parameter estimation was performed using only the intensity samples from the intracranium. As before, the influence of the value of trimming fraction on the performance of unsupervised Bayesian-classification based segmentation was analyzed using DSC.

As can be seen from the example segmentation in Fig. 6, the performance of the segmentation based on the proposed mixture-parameter estimation was robust and the obtained segmentation maps were close to ground truth. On the contrary, the FAST-TLE mixture-parameter estimates for high values of trimming fraction led to segmentations with significant errors, especially in the region of ventricular CSF (Fig. 6c). Note that in the provided manual segmentation the extracortical CSF was

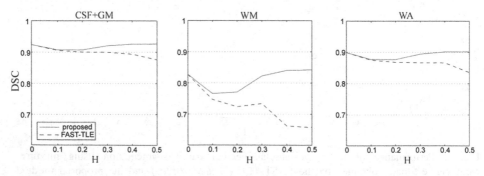

Fig. 7. Performance of the Bayesian-classification based segmentation for combined cerebrospinal fluid and gray matter (CSF+GM), white matter (WM), and volume weighted average (WA), by mixture-parameter estimates of the FAST-TLE in *dashed blue* and the proposed method in *solid red* (Color figure online).

part of the GM class, while the intensity model captured the ventricular and extra-cortical CSF as one component (Fig. 6b). Thus, we evaluate the methods with respect to combined CSF and GM classes, as was proposed in [4]. The results indicate that in average the segmentation performance of the proposed method is more stable than that of FAST-TLE throughout the whole range of tested trimming fractions (Fig. 7).

4 Conclusions

In this paper, we proposed a new method for robust estimation of the parameters of a mixture model for data contaminated by outliers. The method provides a suboptimal solution of the trimmed likelihood maximization, similar to FAST-TLE method. The main advantage of the proposed method is the significance-level based ordering rule of the samples coupled to adaptive trimming fraction, which is re-estimated at each iteration so that the overall trimmed likelihood of the mixture model increases and achieves stable convergence. Note that the trimming fraction corresponds directly to the actual outlier fraction, therefore, the proposed method is more robust to varying fraction of outliers as the popular FAST-TLE method. Our method was tested and compared to FAST-TLE on two-dimensional numerical simulations and three-dimensional synthetic and real brain MR images. The experiments demonstrate that the proposed method has a more predictable behavior as compared to FAST-TLE when applied to mixture-parameter estimation. As the proposed method gives more stable segmentation results over broader range of trimming fraction, the method has great potential to be used for brain tissue segmentation in large-scale multicenter image datasets, where the actual fraction of outliers corresponding to pathological tissues and/or imaging artifacts is unpredictable.

Acknowledgments. This work was supported by the Ministry of Higher Education, Science and Technology under grants L2—4072, P2—0232 and an applied research grant ESRR-07-13-EU.

References

1. Van Leemput, K., Maes, F., Vandermeulen, D., Colchester, A., Suetens, P.: Automated segmentation of multiple sclerosis lesions by model outlier detection. IEEE Trans. Med. Imaging **20**, 677–688 (2001)
2. Garcia-Lorenzo, D., Prima, S., Arnold, D.L., Collins, D.L., Barillot, C.: Trimmed-likelihood estimation for focal lesions and tissue segmentation in multisequence MRI for multiple sclerosis. IEEE Trans. Med. Imaging **30**, 1455–1467 (2011)
3. Nguyen, T.M., Wu, Q.M.J.: Robust student's-t mixture model with spatial constraints and its application in medical image segmentation. IEEE Trans. Med. Imaging **31**, 103–116 (2012)
4. Roy, S., Carass, A., Bazin, P.-L., Resnick, S., Prince, J.L.: Consistent segmentation using a Rician classifier. Med. Image Anal. **16**, 524–535 (2012)
5. Dempster, A.P., Laird, N.M., Rubin, D.B.: Maximum likelihood from incomplete data via the EM algorithm. J. Roy. Stat. Soc. B **39**, 1–38 (1977)

6. Hodge, V.J., Austin, J.: A survey of outlier detection methodologies. Artif. Intell. Rev. **22**, 85–126 (2004)
7. Neykov, N., Filzmoser, P., Dimova, R., Neytchev, P.: Robust fitting of mixtures using the trimmed likelihood estimator. Comput. Stat. Data Anal. **52**, 299–308 (2007)
8. Aït-Ali, L.S., Prima, S., Hellier, P., Carsin, B., Edan, G., Barillot, C.: STREM: a robust multidimensional parametric method to segment MS lesions in MRI. In: Duncan, J., Gerig, G. (eds.) MICCAI 2005. LNCS, vol. 3749, pp. 409–416. Springer, Heidelberg (2005)
9. Bricq, S., Collet, C., Armspach, J.: MS lesion segmentation based on hidden Markov chains. Presented at the Grand Challenge Workshop: Multiple Sclerosis Lesion Segmentation Challenge (2008)
10. Neykov, N.M., Filzmoser, P., Neytchev, P.N.: Robust joint modeling of mean and dispersion through trimming. Comput. Stat. Data Anal. **56**, 34–48 (2012)
11. Otsu, N.: A threshold selection method from gray-level histograms. IEEE Trans. Syst. Man Cybern. **9**, 62–66 (1979)
12. Kwan, R.K.-S., Evans, A.C., Pike, G.B.: MRI simulation-based evaluation of image-processing and classification methods. IEEE Trans. Med. Imaging **18**, 1085–1097 (1999)
13. Dice, L.: Measures of the amount of ecologic association between species. Ecology **26**, 297–302 (1945)
14. Center for Morphometric Analysis (CMA). http://www.cma.mgh.harvard.edu/ibsr/

White Matter Supervoxel Segmentation by Axial DP-Means Clustering

Ryan P. Cabeen[✉] and David H. Laidlaw

Computer Science Department, Brown University, Providence, RI, USA
{cabeen,dhl}@cs.brown.edu

Abstract. A powerful aspect of diffusion MR imaging is the ability to reconstruct fiber orientations in brain white matter; however, the application of traditional learning algorithms is challenging due to the directional nature of the data. In this paper, we present an algorithmic approach to clustering such spatial and orientation data and apply it to brain white matter supervoxel segmentation. This approach is an extension of the DP-means algorithm to support axial data, and we present its theoretical connection to probabilistic models, including the Gaussian and Watson distributions. We evaluate our method with the analysis of synthetic data and an application to diffusion tensor atlas segmentation. We find our approach to be efficient and effective for the automatic extraction of regions of interest that respect the structure of brain white matter. The resulting supervoxel segmentation could be used to map regional anatomical changes in clinical studies or serve as a domain for more complex modeling.

Keywords: Diffusion tensor imaging · Atlasing · Segmentation · Parcellation · White matter · Clustering · Supervoxels · Bregman divergence · Directional statistics

1 Introduction and Related Work

Diffusion MR imaging enables the quantitative measurement of water molecule diffusion, which exhibits anisotropy in brain white matter due to axonal morphometry and coherence. Consequently, the orientation of fibers passing through a voxel can be estimated from the diffusion signal, allowing the local analysis of tissue or more global analysis of fiber bundles. Methods from computer vision and machine learning offer many opportunities to understand the structure captured by diffusion MRI; however, the directional nature of the data poses a challenge to traditional methods.

A successful approach for dealing with this directional data has been probabilistic models on the sphere; the two most common being the von Mises-Fisher and Watson distributions. The Watson distinguishes itself by being defined for axial variables, that is, points on the sphere with anti-podal equivalence. These models have been known in the statistics community for decades and

B. Menze et al. (Eds.): MCV 2013, LNCS 8331, pp. 95–104, 2014.
DOI: 10.1007/978-3-319-05530-5_10, © Springer International Publishing Switzerland 2014

have applications to a number of disciplines, including geophysics, chemistry, genomics, and information retrieval [16]. Recently, there has been increasing interest in exploring directional mixture models for neuroimage analysis [6,10]. They can be computationally challenging, however, as their normalization constants have no closed form and require either strong assumptions [11] or approximations [12].

This problem is not unique to directional data, however, and there has been much work to develop efficient and scalable alternatives to probabilistic models. Some success in this area applies to the exponential families, which constitute most distributions in use today. Banerjee et al. made a powerful finding which established a bijection between the exponential families and Bregman divergences. They also explored the asymptotic relationship between mixture models and hard clustering algorithms [2]. These hard clustering algorithms tend to be more efficient, scalable, and easy to implement, at the cost of some flexibility in data modeling. We build on these ideas to derive hard clustering for data that has both spatial and directional components. Our approach extends this idea to axial data by considering the Bregman divergergence of the Watson distribution [12]. We employ additional prior work in this area that derived the DP-means algorithm from the asymptotic limit of a Dirichlet process mixture [5,7], providing a data-driven way to select the number of clusters. We define our segmentation from the hard clustering of voxels, so we use the terms interchangably for the rest of the paper.

Segmentation algorithms offer an opportunity to study neuroanatomy in an automated way, reducing the cost of manual delineation of anatomical structures. We consider voxelwise segmentation, as opposed to methods that cluster curves extracted by tractography. One common application of the voxelwise approach is the segmentation of the thalamic nuclei, which has been achieved by mean shift analysis, spectral clustering, level-sets, and modified k-means [17]. The work of Weigell et al. is most similar to the approach we propose, as they apply a k-means-like algorithm, modified to operate in the joint spatial-tensor domain. In contrast, we include optimization for model complexity, instead of selecting a fixed number of clusters as in k-means. We also operate on the fiber orientation, instead of the full tensor, a reasonable simplification for the segmentation of white matter, which is more anisotropic than gray matter.

We consider a segmentation of whole brain white matter in which numerous small and homogenous regions (or supervoxels) are extracted, an approach that is similar to superpixel segmentation in the computer vision literature [13]. Superpixels have been found to offer both a more natural representation of images compared to pixels and a simpler domain for more complex models [9]. In the field of biomedical imaging, this idea has recently been successfully applied to spectral label fusion [15], cellular imaging [8] and fiber orientation distribution-based segmentation [3], to which our work bears similarity.

The rest of the paper is as follows. First, we review the exponential families and their relation to Bregman divergences. We then present the models and Bregman divergences of the Gaussian and Watson distributions. From these, we derive an axial DP-means algorithm that clusters voxels in the joint spatial-axial domain. Finally, we present an evaluation with synthetic data and an application to diffusion tensor atlas white matter supervoxel segmentation.

2 Methods

2.1 Exponential Families and Bregman Divergences

In this section, we review the exponential families, its relationship to Bregman divergences, and applications of this $\hat{p}$ divergence to clustering problems.

A parameteric family of distributions is considered exponential when members have a density of the following form [1]:

$$P_G(\mathbf{x}|\boldsymbol{\theta}) = P_0(\mathbf{x}) \exp(<\boldsymbol{\theta}, \mathbf{x}> -G(\boldsymbol{\theta})) \qquad (1)$$

where $\boldsymbol{\theta}$ is the natural (or canonical) parameter, $\mathbf{x}$ is the sufficient statistic, $G(\boldsymbol{\theta})$ is the cumulant (or log-partition) function, and $P_0(\mathbf{x})$ is the carrier measure. The exponential families have a variety of useful properties, but here we consider their relation to Bregman divergences, a measure which can be interpreted as relative entropy. Banerjee et al. showed a bijection between the exponential families and Bregman divergences [2], and consequently, the divergence corresponding to a given member of the exponential family can be defined from the cumulant [1]:

$$\Delta_G(\hat{\boldsymbol{\theta}}, \boldsymbol{\theta}) = G(\hat{\boldsymbol{\theta}}) - G(\boldsymbol{\theta}) - <\hat{\boldsymbol{\theta}} - \boldsymbol{\theta}, \nabla_{\boldsymbol{\theta}} G(\boldsymbol{\theta})> \qquad (2)$$

This result gives a probabilistic interpretation to many distance measures. In particular, a number of hard clustering objectives may be expressed in terms of Bregman divergences associated with exponential mixture models, showing a relationship between soft and hard clustering algorithms [5]. This result can also be used to derive hard clustering algorithms for directional data, as described in the following sections.

2.2 Gaussian and Watson Distributions

We now consider two probabilistic models for our data, namely the Gaussian and Watson distributions, which represent spatial and axial data, respectively. For each distribution, we show the form of their distribution, derive their associated Bregman divergences, and discuss their relationship to hard clustering algorithms in the literature.

The isotropic Gaussian distribution is defined on $\mathbb{R}^n$ and is commonly used to represent spatial data. Its probability density $\mathcal{N}$ and associated Bregman divergence $D_{\mathcal{N}}$ are given by:

$$\mathcal{N}(\mathbf{p}|\mathbf{q}, \sigma^2) = \frac{1}{(2\pi\sigma^2)^{n/2}} \exp\left(-\frac{1}{2\sigma^2}||\mathbf{p} - \mathbf{q}||^2\right) \qquad (3)$$

$$D_{\mathcal{N}}(\hat{\mathbf{p}}, \mathbf{p}) = \frac{1}{2\sigma^2}||\hat{\mathbf{p}} - \mathbf{p}||^2 \qquad (4)$$

given input positions $\mathbf{p}, \hat{\mathbf{p}} \in \mathbb{R}^n$, mean position $\mathbf{q} \in \mathbb{R}^n$, and constant variance parameter $\sigma^2 > 0$. The associated Bregman divergence $D_{\mathcal{N}}$ is the scaled Euclidean distance between two positions, an observation which gives a probabilistic interpretation to the k-means and DP-means algorithms, which are asymptotic limits of Gaussian mixture and Dirichlet process mixture models, respectively [7].

The Watson distribution is analogous to a Gaussian but defined on the hypersphere $S^{n-1} \subset \mathbb{R}^n$ with anti-podal symmetry, i.e. $\mathbf{d} \sim -\mathbf{d}$. This structure is well-suited to diffusion MR, for which a sign is not associated with the diffusion direction. Samples from this distribution are often called axial variables to distinguish them from spherical data without symmetry. Its probability density W and associated Bregman divergence D_W are given by:

$$W(\mathbf{d}|\mathbf{v}, \kappa) = \frac{\Gamma(n/2)}{(2\pi)^{n/2} M(\frac{1}{2}, \frac{n}{2}, \kappa)} \exp\left(\kappa \left(\mathbf{v}^T \mathbf{d}\right)^2\right) \tag{5}$$

$$D_W(\hat{\mathbf{d}}, \mathbf{d}) = \kappa \frac{M(\frac{1}{2}, \frac{n}{2}, \kappa)}{M'(\frac{1}{2}, \frac{n}{2}, \kappa)} \left(1 - \left(\hat{\mathbf{d}}^T \mathbf{d}\right)^2\right) \tag{6}$$

for input axial directions $\mathbf{d}, \hat{\mathbf{d}} \in S^{n-1}$, mean axial direction $\mathbf{v} \in S^{n-1}$, and Kummer's confluent hypergeometric function $M(a, b, z)$. We also assume a constant and positive concentration parameter $\kappa > 0$. The associated Bregman divergence D_W is then a scaled cosine-squared dissimilarity measure, which is equivalent to the measure used for diametrical clustering—the asymptotic limit of a mixture of Watsons [4,12]. The Bregman divergences for the Gaussian and Watson distributions can then be used to define hard clustering algorithms, which we'll describe next.

2.3 Hard Clustering

We now present an objective function for clustering axial data and an iterative algorithm for optimizing it. In particular, this approach is a hard clustering algorithm that behaves similarly to a Dirichlet process (DP) mixture model learned with Gibbs sampling, as a result of recent work on small-variance asymptotic analysis of the exponential family and Bregman divergences by Jiang et al. [5]. We apply their work to our case of spatial and axial data, which is assumed to be modeled jointly by the Gaussian and Watson distributions.

For imaging applications, segmentation is often performed in the joint spatial-intensity space. A common application is superpixel segmentation, which provides a domain for image understanding that is both more simple and natural than the original pixel domain [9]. This is also the case for diffusion MR, where we want to segment voxels based on both proximity and fiber orientation similarity, perhaps to aid more complex anatomical modeling [3]. This motivates the development of a clustering algorithm that accounts for these two aspects, which we achieve by the linear combination of the Bregman divergences presented in the previous section. The resulting objective function E can be defined similarly to the DP-means algorithm:

$$E = \sum_{k=1}^{K} \sum_{(\mathbf{p},\mathbf{d}) \in l_k} D_{\mathcal{N}}(\mathbf{p}, \mathbf{q}_k) + D_W(\mathbf{d}, \mathbf{v}_k) + \lambda K \tag{7}$$

$$E = \sum_{k=1}^{K} \sum_{(\mathbf{p},\mathbf{d}) \in l_k} \alpha \|\mathbf{p} - \mathbf{q}_k\|^2 + \beta \left(1 - \left(\mathbf{v}_k^T \mathbf{d}\right)^2\right) + \lambda K \tag{8}$$

where l_k is the set of voxels in the k-th cluster, λ is a cluster-penalty term that controls model complexity, and the parameters α and β control the relative contributions of the spatial and axial terms to the total cost. These parameters have probabilistic interpretations, where λ relates to the Dirichlet process mixture prior, and α and β relate to the Gaussian σ and Watson κ, respectively.

A procedure to minimize this objective is presented in Algorithm 1. In a modification of the DP-means algorithm [7], the assignment step measures distance by the linear combination of divergences. In the update step, the spatial cluster center $\mathbf{q}_c$ is computed by the Euclidean average. The axial cluster center $\mathbf{v}_c$ is computed by the maximum likelihood approach of Schwartzman et al. [11], where dyadic tensors are computed by the outer product of each axial variable and the mean axial direction is found from the principal eigenvector of the mean tensor, as shown by the *prineig* function.

Algorithm 1. joint spatial-axial DP-means clustering

Input:
    $(\mathbf{p}_1, \mathbf{d}_1), ..., (\mathbf{p}_N, \mathbf{d}_N)$: input position/axial direction pairs,
    α, β, λ: objective weighting parameters
Output:
    K: number of clusters, $L_1, ..., L_N$: labels,
    $(\mathbf{q}_1, \mathbf{v}_1), ..., (\mathbf{q}_K, \mathbf{v}_K)$: cluster centers

Initialize: $K \leftarrow 1$, $\mathbf{q}_1 \leftarrow \sum_i \mathbf{p}_i / N$, $\mathbf{v}_1 \leftarrow prineig\left(\sum_i \mathbf{d}_i \mathbf{d}_i^T / N\right)$
while *not converged* **do**
    Assign cluster labels:
    for *i=1* **to** *N* **do**
        for *j=1* **to** *K* **do**
            $D_{ij} \leftarrow \alpha \|\mathbf{p}_i - \mathbf{q}_j\|^2 + \beta \left(1 - \left(d_i^T \mathbf{v}_j\right)^2\right)$
        if $\min_j D_{ij} > \lambda$ **then**
            $K \leftarrow K + 1$, $\mathbf{q}_K \leftarrow \mathbf{p}_i$, $\mathbf{v}_K \leftarrow d_i$, $L_i \leftarrow K$
        else
            $L_i \leftarrow \operatorname{argmin}_j D_{ij}$
    Update cluster centers:
    for *j=1* **to** *K* **do**
        $\mathbf{q}_j \leftarrow \left(\sum_i \delta(j, L_i) \mathbf{p}_i\right) / \sum_i \delta(j, L_i)$
        $\mathbf{v}_j \leftarrow prineig\left(\left(\sum_i \delta(j, L_i) \mathbf{d}_i \mathbf{d}_i^T\right) / \sum_i \delta(j, L_i)\right)$
return

---

3   Experiments and Results

3.1   Synthetic Data

In our first experiment, we investigate the choice of the cluster penalty parameter λ by synthesizing axial data and testing performance of the axial DP-means algorithm across varying numbers and sizes of clusters. Here, we ignore the spatial component and only test the relationship between λ and the axial clustering. The number of clusters N ranged from 3 to 10 and were generated by sampling a Gaussian and normalizing with "size" σ ranging from 0.1 to 0.3. We evaluated ground truth agreement with the adjusted mutual information score (AMI) [14], a statistical measure of similarity between clusterings that accounts for chance groupings and takes a maximum value of one when clusterings are equivalent.

For a constant number of clusters, we found the optimal choice of λ increased with cluster size σ. For a constant cluster size σ, we found the optimal λ to be relatively stable across variable numbers of clusters N. In Fig. 1, we show examples of the clustering for the two conditions. In Fig. 2, we show plots of the relationship between the AMI and λ. We found our implementation to converge in fewer than 20 iterations on average. All cases except one found the correct number of clusters for the optimal λ. This could be due to the presence of local minima, an issue that could possibly be addressed with a randomized initialization scheme and restarts.

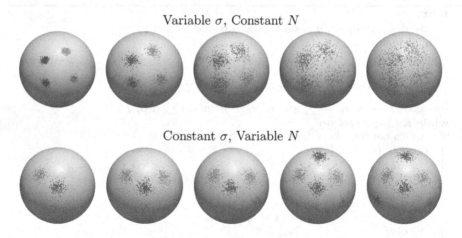

Fig. 1. First experiment: visualizations of the synthetic axial data and the optimal clusterings computed from the proposed method. The top shows results for variable cluster size $\sigma = \{0.05, 0.0875, 0.125, 0.1625, 0.2\}$, and constant number of clusters $N = 4$. The bottom shows results for constant cluster size $\sigma = 0.10$, and variable number of clusters $N = \{3, 4, 5, 6, 7\}$. The bottom right shows a single mislabeled cluster, possibly caused by finding a local minima in the optimization.

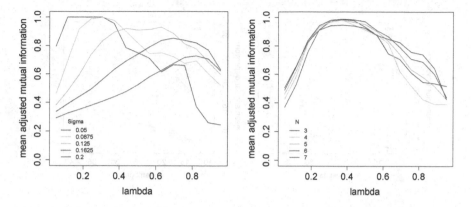

Fig. 2. First experiment: clustering performance as a function of cluster penalty para-meter $\lambda \in [0, 1]$ given ground truth generated with cluster size σ, and number of clus-ters N, which are visualized in Fig. 1. We measured the adjusted mutual information (AMI), a statistical measure takes a maximal value when clusterings are equivalent. Shown are plots of the AMI vs. λ for two conditions. The first tested with variable $\sigma = \{0.05, 0.0875, 0.125, 0.1625, 0.2\}$ and constant $N = 4$. The second tested with con-stant $\sigma = 0.10$ and variable $N = \{3, 4, 5, 6, 7\}$. These results indicate that the optimal λ depends more on σ than N, suggesting that performance may depend on the noise level and may dimishish when differing clusters sizes are present. Also note that the maximum AMI decreases with increasing σ, which may be due to cluster overlap or over-sensitivity in the AMI measure.

3.2   White Matter Segmentation

In our second experiment, we apply the axial DP-means algorithm to the super-voxel segmentation of brain white matter in a diffusion tensor atlas. We used the IXI aging brain atlas, which was constructed by deformable tensor-based registration with DTI-TK [19]. White matter was extracted by thresholding the fractional anisotropy map at a value of 0.2, which excludes white matter voxels with complex fiber configurations that are not accurately represented by tensors.

We then performed white matter segmentation of the remaining voxels with the joint spatial-axial DP-means algorithm. For each voxel, the spatial com-ponent was taken to be the voxel center and the directional component was taken to be the principal direction of the voxel's tensor. We found several struc-tures which were spatially disconnected but given the same label, for example, the bilateral cingulum bundles, which are both close and similarly oriented. To account for this, we finally performed connected components labeling using an efficient two-pass procedure [18].

We investigated the effect of λ and β (holding α constant) by measuring the mean cluster orientation dispersion and cluster volume. We found that as λ was increased, both the volume and angular dispersion increased. As β increased, we observed decreased cluster volume and angular dispersion. These results are shown in the plots of Fig. 3. We also generated visualizations from a segmentation

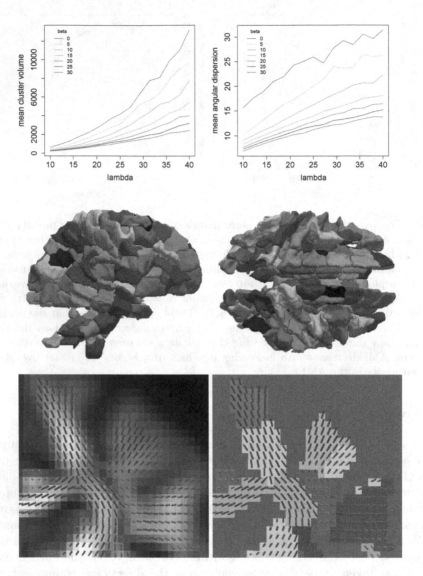

Fig. 3. Second experiment: white matter supervoxel segmentation by axial DP-means clustering. The top row shows mean cluster volume (mm^3) and mean cluster angular dispersion (degrees) as a function of cluster penalty $\lambda \in [10, 40]$ and axial weighting $\beta \in [0, 30]$. We found increasing λ also increased the volume and dispersion, while increasing β reduced the volume and dispersion. The middle and bottom rows show an example result given $\lambda = 25$ and $\beta = 15$. The middle shows boundary surfaces of the regions, which illustrates the symmetry and separation of gyral and deep white matter. The bottom shows a partial coronal slice with the fractional anisotropy (left) and computed segmentation (right), whish shows region boundaries that match known anatomical interfaces, such as the corpus callosum/cingulum bundle and corona radiata/superior longitudinal fasciculus.

with $\lambda = 25$ and $\beta = 15$, which are shown in Fig. 3. From slice views, we found the segmentation to reflect known anatomical boundaries, such as the cingulum/corpus callosum and corona radiata/superior longitudinal fasciculus. By overlaying fiber models, we see the region boundaries tended to coincide with large changes in fiber orientation. From an boundary surface rendering, we found lateral symmetry and a separation of gyral white matter from deeper white matter. Our serial implementation on a 2.3 GHz Intel i5 ran in several minutes and converged in 125 iterations.

4 Discussion and Conclusions

In this paper, we presented an efficient approach to hard clustering of spatial and axial data that is effective for segmenting brain white matter. This algorithm has a probabilistic interpretation that relates its objective to the Bregman divergences of the Gaussian and Watson distributions. Through our experiments, we first found the parameter λ to be more affected by cluster size σ than the number of clusters N. This may suggest the need to account for noise level when selecting λ and possible limitations when applied to datasets with clusters of heterogeneous size. In our second experiment, we found our approach to efficiently perform white matter atlas segmentation, producing regions that respect anatomical boundies in white matter structure. We also found considerable variablility across different hyperparameters. On one hand, this offers fine-grained control of region size, but it also suggests that a comparison with a simpler k-means type approach could be valuable. A limitation is the restriction of this approach to single fiber voxels and extensions to multiple fibers could be valuable. This could be possibly used with other methods for reconstucting fiber orientations, such as orientation distribution function (ODF) and fiber orientation distribution (FOD) approaches.

This method may also aid several aspects of clinical studies of white matter. The resulting segmentation could provide automatically defined regions-of-interest for clinical study, similar to voxel-based population studies of neurological disease. This approach may also offers a domain for more efficient inference of complex anatomical models, such as graph-based methods for measuring brain connectivity. One interesting extension would generalize the clustering objective to include variable concentration κ, which may enable more sensitive segmentation for diffusion models that account for fiber orientation dispersion in each voxel. In conclusion, we find this approach to be an efficient and valuable tool for segmenting white matter with a desirable probabilistic interpretation and a number of applications to brain connectivity mapping.

References

1. Azoury, K.S., Warmuth, M.K.: Relative loss bounds for on-line density estimation with the exponential family of distributions. Mach. Learn. **43**(3), 211–246 (2001)

2. Banerjee, A., Merugu, S., Dhillon, I.S., Ghosh, J.: Clustering with Bregman divergences. J. Mach. Learn. Res. **6**, 1705–1749 (2005)
3. Bloy, L., Ingalhalikar, M., Eavani, H., Schultz, R.T., Roberts, T.P., Verma, R.: White matter atlas generation using HARDI based automated parcellation. Neuroimage **59**(4), 4055–4063 (2012)
4. Dhillon, I.S., Marcotte, E.M., Roshan, U.: Diametrical clustering for identifying anti-correlated gene clusters. Bioinformatics **19**(13), 1612–1619 (2003)
5. Jiang, K., Kulis, B., Jordan, M.: Small-variance asymptotics for exponential family Dirichlet process mixture models. In: NIPS 2012 (2012)
6. Kaden, E., Kruggel, F.: Nonparametric Bayesian inference of the fiber orientation distribution from diffusion-weighted MR images. Med. Image Anal. **16**(4), 876–888 (2012)
7. Kulis, B., Jordan, M.I.: Revisiting k-means: new algorithms via Bayesian nonparametrics. In: ICML-12, pp. 513–520 (2012)
8. Lucchi, A., Smith, K., Achanta, R., Lepetit, V., Fua, P.: A fully automated approach to segmentation of irregularly shaped cellular structures in EM images. In: Jiang, T., Navab, N., Pluim, J.P.W., Viergever, M.A. (eds.) MICCAI 2010, Part II. LNCS, vol. 6362, pp. 463–471. Springer, Heidelberg (2010)
9. Mori, G.: Guiding model search using segmentation. In: ICCV 2005, vol. 2, pp. 1417–1423 (2005)
10. Rathi, Y., Michailovich, O., Shenton, M.E., Bouix, S.: Directional functions for orientation distribution estimation. Med. Image Anal. **13**(3), 432–444 (2009)
11. Schwartzman, A., Dougherty, R.F., Taylor, J.E.: Cross-subject comparison of principal diffusion direction maps. Magnet. Reson. Med. **53**(6), 1423–1431 (2005)
12. Sra, S., Karp, D.: The multivariate Watson distribution: maximum-likelihood estimation and other aspects. J. Multivar. Anal. **114**, 256–269 (2013)
13. Veksler, O., Boykov, Y., Mehrani, P.: Superpixels and supervoxels in an energy optimization framework. In: Daniilidis, K., Maragos, P., Paragios, N. (eds.) ECCV 2010, Part V. LNCS, vol. 6315, pp. 211–224. Springer, Heidelberg (2010)
14. Vinh, N.X., Epps, J., Bailey, J.: Information theoretic measures for clusterings comparison: variants, properties, normalization and correction for chance. J. Mach. Learn. Res. **11**, 2837–2854 (2010)
15. Wachinger, C., Golland, P.: Spectral label fusion. In: Ayache, N., Delingette, H., Golland, P., Mori, K. (eds.) MICCAI 2012, Part III. LNCS, vol. 7512, pp. 410–417. Springer, Heidelberg (2012)
16. Watson, G.S.: Statistics on spheres, vol. 6. Wiley, New York (1983)
17. Wiegell, M.R., Tuch, D.S., Larsson, H.B., Wedeen, V.J.: Automatic segmentation of thalamic nuclei from diffusion tensor magnetic resonance imaging. Neuroimage **19**(2), 391–401 (2003)
18. Wu, K., Otoo, E., Suzuki, K.: Optimizing two-pass connected-component labeling algorithms. Pattern Anal. Appl. **12**(2), 117–135 (2009)
19. Zhang, H., Yushkevich, P.A., Rueckert, D., Gee, J.C.: A computational white matter atlas for aging with surface-based representation of fasciculi. In: Fischer, B., Dawant, B., Lorenz, C. (eds.) WBIR 2010. LNCS, vol. 6204, pp. 83–90. Springer, Heidelberg (2010)

Semantic Context Forests for Learning-Based Knee Cartilage Segmentation in 3D MR Images

Quan Wang[1,2(✉)], Dijia Wu[1], Le Lu[1], Meizhu Liu[1],
Kim L. Boyer[2], and Shaohua Kevin Zhou[1]

[1] Siemens Corporate Research, Princeton, NJ 08540, USA
wangq10@rpi.edu
[2] Rensselaer Polytechnic Institute, Troy, NY 12180, USA

Abstract. The automatic segmentation of human knee cartilage from 3D MR images is a useful yet challenging task due to the thin sheet structure of the cartilage with diffuse boundaries and inhomogeneous intensities. In this paper, we present an iterative multi-class learning method to segment the femoral, tibial and patellar cartilage simultaneously, which effectively exploits the spatial contextual constraints between bone and cartilage, and also between different cartilages. First, based on the fact that the cartilage grows in only certain area of the corresponding bone surface, we extract the distance features of not only to the surface of the bone, but more informatively, to the densely registered anatomical landmarks on the bone surface. Second, we introduce a set of iterative discriminative classifiers that at each iteration, probability comparison features are constructed from the class confidence maps derived by previously learned classifiers. These features automatically embed the semantic context information between different cartilages of interest. Validated on a total of 176 volumes from the Osteoarthritis Initiative (OAI) dataset, the proposed approach demonstrates high robustness and accuracy of segmentation in comparison with existing state-of-the-art MR cartilage segmentation methods.

1 Introduction

The quantitative analysis of knee cartilage is advantageous for the study of cartilage morphology and physiology. In particular, it is an important prerequisite for the clinical assessment and surgical planning of the cartilage diseases, such as knee osteoarthritis which is characterized as the cartilage deterioration and a prevalent cause of disability among elderly population. As the leading imaging modality used for articular cartilage quantification [1], magnetic resonance (MR) imaging provides direct and noninvasive visualization of the whole knee joint including the soft cartilage tissues (Fig. 1c). However, automatic segmentation of the cartilage tissues from MR images, which is required for accurate and reproducible quantitative cartilage measures, still remains an open problem because of the inhomogeneity, small size, low tissue contrast, and shape irregularity of the cartilage.

B. Menze et al. (Eds.): MCV 2013, LNCS 8331, pp. 105–115, 2014.
DOI: 10.1007/978-3-319-05530-5_11, © Springer International Publishing Switzerland 2014

An earlier endeavor on this problem is Folkesson *et al.*'s voxel classification approach [2], which runs an approximate kNN classifier on voxel intensity and absolute position based features. However, due to the overlap of intensity distribution between cartilage and other tissues such as menisci and muscles, as well as the variability of the cartilage locations from scan to scan, the performance of this method is limited. More recently, Vincent *et al.* have developed a knee joint segmentation approach based on active appearance model (AAM), which captures the statistics of both object shape and image cues. Though promising results are reported in [3], the search for the initial model pose parameter can be very time consuming even if a coarse to fine searching strategy is used.

Given the strong spatial relation between the cartilages and bones in the knee joint, most proposed cartilage segmentation methods are based on a framework that each bone is segmented first in the knee joint [4–6], which is usually easier than direct cartilage segmentation because the bones are much larger in size with more regular shapes. Fripp *et al.* segment the bones based on 3D active shape model (ASM) incorporating the cartilage thickness statistics, and the outer cartilage boundary is then determined by examining the intensity profile along the normal to the bone surface, while being constrained by the cartilage thickness model [4]. In Yin's work [5], the volume of interest containing the bones and cartilages is first detected using a learning-based approach, then the bones and cartilages are jointly segmented by solving an optimal multi-surface detection problem via multi-column graph cuts [7]. Lee *et al.* employ a constrained branch-and-mincut method with shape priors to obtain the bone surface, and then segment the cartilage with MRF optimization based on local shape and appearance information [6]. In spite of the differences, these approaches all require classification of bone surface voxels into bone cartilage interface (BCI) and non-BCI, which is an important intermediate step to determine the search space or impose prior constraint for cartilage segmentation. Therefore, any classification error of BCI will probably propagate to the final cartilage segmentation result.

In this paper, we present a fully automatic learning-based voxel classification method for cartilage segmentation. It also requires pre-segmentation of corresponding bones in the knee joint. However, the new approach does not rely on explicit classification of BCI. Instead, we construct distance features from each voxel to a large number of anatomical landmarks on the surface of the bones to capture the spatial relation between the cartilages and bones. By removing the intermediate step of BCI extraction, the whole framework is simplified and classification error propagation can be avoided.

Besides the connection between the cartilages and bones, strong spatial relation also exists among different cartilages which is more often overlooked in earlier approaches. For example, the femoral cartilage is always above the tibial cartilage and two cartilages touch each other in the region where two bones slide over each other during joint movements. To utilize this constraint, we introduce the iterative discriminative classification that at each iteration, the multi-class probability maps obtained by previous classifiers are used to extract semantic context features. In particular, we compare the probabilities at positions with random shift and compute the difference. These features, which we name as the random shift probability difference (RSPD) features, are more computationally efficient and more flexible for different range of context compared to the calculation of probability statistics at fixed relative positions [8,9].

2   Review of Bone Segmentation

In this work, we employ a learning-based bone segmentation approach which has shown the efficiency and effectiveness in different medical image segmentation problems [10,11]. We represent the shape of a bone by a closed triangle mesh $\mathcal{M}$. Given a number of training volumes with manual bone annotations, we use the coherent point drift algorithm (CPD) [12] to find anatomical correspondences of the mesh points and thereof construct the statistical shape models with mean shape $\overline{\mathcal{M}}$ [13]. As shown in Fig. 1a, the whole bone segmentation framework comprises three steps.

1. Pose Estimation: For a volume $\mathcal{V}$, the bone is first localized by searching for the (sub-)optimal pose parameters $(\hat{t}, \hat{r}, \hat{s})$, i.e., the translation, rotation and anisotropic scaling, using the marginal space learning (MSL) [11]:

$$(\hat{t}, \hat{r}, \hat{s}) \approx (\arg \max_t P(t|\mathcal{V}), \arg \max_r P(r|\mathcal{V}, \hat{t}), \arg \max_s P(s|\mathcal{V}, \hat{t}, \hat{r})), \quad (1)$$

   and the shape is initialized by linearly transforming the mean shape $\overline{\mathcal{M}}$.
2. Model Deformation: At this stage, the shape is repeatedly deformed to fit the boundary and projected to the variation subspace until convergence.
3. Boundary Refinement: To further improve the segmentation accuracy, we use the random walks algorithm [14] to refine the bone boundary (see Table 1 and Fig. 4 for results) and employ the CPD algorithm to obtain anatomically equivalent landmarks on the refined bone surface.

3   Cartilage Classification

Given all three knee bones being segmented, we first extract a band of interest within a maximum distance threshold from each of the bone surface, and only classify voxels in the band of interest to simplify the training and testing by removing irrelevant negative voxels.

3.1   Feature Extraction

For each voxel with spatial coordinate $\mathbf{x}$, we construct a number of base features which can be categorized into three subsets.

Intensity Features include the voxel intensity and its gradient magnitude, respectively: $f_1(\mathbf{x}) = I(\mathbf{x})$, $f_2(\mathbf{x}) = ||\nabla I(\mathbf{x})||$.

Distance Features measure the signed Euclidean distances from each voxel to different knee bone boundaries: $f_3(\mathbf{x}) = d_F(\mathbf{x})$, $f_4(\mathbf{x}) = d_T(\mathbf{x})$, $f_5(\mathbf{x}) = d_P(\mathbf{x})$,

Table 1. The Dice similarity coefficient (DSC) of bone segmentation results before and after random walks (3-fold cross validation on 176 OAI volumes)

	Femur DSC (%)	Tibia DSC (%)	Patella DSC (%)
Before RW	92.37 ± 1.58	94.64 ± 1.18	92.07 ± 1.47
After RW	94.86 ± 1.85	95.96 ± 1.64	94.31 ± 2.15

where d_F is the signed distance to the femur, d_T to tibia, and d_P to patella. Then we have their linear combinations:

$$f_{6/7}(\mathbf{x}) = d_F(\mathbf{x}) \pm d_T(\mathbf{x}), \qquad f_{8/9}(\mathbf{x}) = d_F(\mathbf{x}) \pm d_P(\mathbf{x}). \qquad (2)$$

These features are useful because the sum features f_6 and f_8 measure whether voxel $\mathbf{x}$ locates within the narrow space between two bones, and the difference features f_7 and f_9 measure which bone it is closer to. Figure 3b shows how f_6 and f_7 in addition to intensity feature f_1 separate tibial cartilage from femoral and patellar cartilages.

Given the prior knowledge that the cartilage can only grow in certain area on the bone surface, it is useful for the cartilage segmentation to not only know how close the voxel is to the bone surface, but also where it is anatomically. Therefore we define the distance features to the densely registered landmarks on the bone surface as described in Sect. 2: $f_{10}(\mathbf{x}, \zeta) = ||\mathbf{x} - \mathbf{z}_\zeta||$, where $\mathbf{z}_\zeta$ is the spatial coordinate of the ζth landmark of all bone mesh points. ζ is randomly generated in training due to the great number of mesh points available (Fig. 3a).

Context Features compare the intensity of the current voxel $\mathbf{x}$ and another voxel $\mathbf{x} + \mathbf{u}$ with random offset $\mathbf{u}$: $f_{11}(\mathbf{x}, \mathbf{u}) = I(\mathbf{x} + \mathbf{u}) - I(\mathbf{x})$, where $\mathbf{u}$ is a random offset vector. This subset of features, named as random shift intensity difference (RSID) features in this paper, capture the context information in different ranges by randomly generating a large number of different values of $\mathbf{u}$ from a uniform distribution in training. They were earlier used to solve pose classification [15] and keypoint recognition [16] problems.

3.2   Iterative Semantic Context Forests

In this paper, we present a multi-pass iterative classification method to automatically exploit the semantic context for multiple object segmentation problems. In each pass, the generated probability maps will be used to extract the context embedded features to enhance the classification performance of the next pass. Figure 1d shows a 2-pass iterative classification framework with the random forests [15–20] selected as the base classifier for each pass. However, the method can be extended to more iterations with the use of other discriminative classifiers.

Semantic Context Features. After each pass of the classification, the probability maps are generated and used to extract semantic context features as

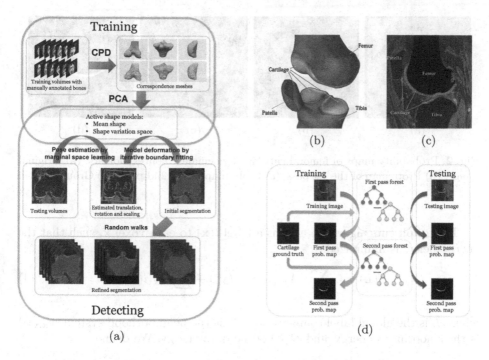

Fig. 1. (a) The bone segmentation framework. (b) 3D anatomy of knee joint. (c) Example of a 2D MR slice [6]. (d) The semantic context forests diagram.

defined below: $f_{12}(\mathbf{x}) = P_F(\mathbf{x})$, $f_{13}(\mathbf{x}) = P_T(\mathbf{x})$, $f_{14}(\mathbf{x}) = P_P(\mathbf{x})$, where P_F, P_T and P_P stand for the femoral, tibia and patellar cartilage probability map, respectively. In the same fashion as the RSID features, we compare the probability response of two voxels with random shift:

$$f_{15/16/17}(\mathbf{x}, \mathbf{u}) = P_{F/T/P}(\mathbf{x} + \mathbf{u}) - P_{F/T/P}(\mathbf{x}), \qquad (3)$$

which is called random shift probability difference features (RSPD). RSPD provides semantic context information because the probability map values are directly associated with anatomical labels, rather than original intensity volume.

In Fig. 2, it can be observed that the probability map of the second pass classification is significantly enhanced with much less noisy responses, compared with the first pass.

3.3   Post-processing by Graph Cuts Optimization

After the classification, we finally use the probabilities of being the background and the three cartilages to construct the energy functions and perform multi-label graph cuts [21] to refine the segmentation with smoothness constraints.

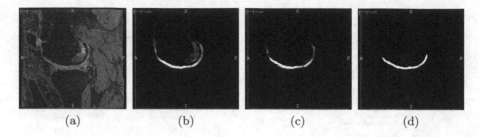

(a)   (b)   (c)   (d)

Fig. 2. Probability maps of femoral cartilage by semantic context forests. (a) Original image. (b) Prob. map of the 1st pass. (c) Prob. map of the 2nd pass. (d) Ground truth.

The graph cuts algorithm assigns a label $l(\mathbf{x})$ to each voxel $\mathbf{x}$, such that the energy below is minimized:

$$E(L) = \sum_{\{\mathbf{x},\mathbf{y}\}\in\mathcal{N}} V_{\mathbf{x},\mathbf{y}}(l(\mathbf{x}),l(\mathbf{y})) + \sum_{\mathbf{x}} D_{\mathbf{x}}(l(\mathbf{x})), \quad (4)$$

where L is the global label configuration, $\mathcal{N}$ is the neighborhood system, $V_{\mathbf{x},\mathbf{y}}(\cdot)$ is the smoothness energy, and $D_{\mathbf{x}}(\cdot)$ is the data energy. We define

$$D_{\mathbf{x}}(l(\mathbf{x})) = -\lambda \ln P_{l(\mathbf{x})}(\mathbf{x}), \quad (5)$$

$$V_{\mathbf{x},\mathbf{y}}(l(\mathbf{x}),l(\mathbf{y})) = \delta_{l(\mathbf{x})\neq l(\mathbf{y})} e^{\frac{(I(\mathbf{x})-I(\mathbf{y}))^2}{2\sigma^2}}. \quad (6)$$

$\delta_{l(\mathbf{x})\neq l(\mathbf{y})}$ takes value 1 when $l(\mathbf{x})$ and $l(\mathbf{y})$ are different labels, and takes value 0 when $l(\mathbf{x}) = l(\mathbf{y})$. $P_{l(\mathbf{x})}(\mathbf{x})$ takes the value $P_F(\mathbf{x})$, $P_T(\mathbf{x})$, $P_P(\mathbf{x})$ or $1 - P_F(\mathbf{x}) - P_T(\mathbf{x}) - P_P(\mathbf{x})$, depending on the label $l(\mathbf{x})$. λ and σ are two parameters. λ specifies the weight of data energy versus smoothness energy, while σ is associated with the image noise [22].

4   Experimental Results

4.1   Dataset and Experiment Settings

The dataset we use in our work is the publicly available Osteoarthritis Initiative (OAI) dataset, which contains both 3D MR images and ground truth cartilage annotations, referred to as "kMRI segmentations (iMorphics)". The sagittal 3D 3T (Tesla) DESS (dual echo steady state) WE (water-excitation) MR images in OAI have high-resolution, good delineation of articular cartilage, fast acquisition time and high SNR. Our dataset consists of 176 volumes from 88 subjects, and belongs to the Progression subcohort, where all subjects show symptoms of OA. Each subject has two volumes scanned in different years. The size of each image volume is $384 \times 384 \times 160$ voxels, and the voxel size is $0.365 \times 0.365 \times 0.7\,\mathrm{mm}^3$.

For the validation, we divide the OAI dataset to three equally-sized subsets: D_1, D_2 and D_3, and perform a three-fold validation. The two volumes from the same subject are always placed in the same subset. For each randomized decision tree, we set the depth of the tree to 18, and train 60 trees in each pass. During training, the number of candidates at each non-leaf node is set to 1000. The dice similarity coefficient (DSC) is used to measure the performance of our method since it is commonly reported in previous literature [2, 4–6, 23].

4.2   Results

First, we compare the frequency of different features that is selected by the classifiers. As shown in Fig. 3c, RSID, RSPD and the distance to dense landmarks are very informative features to embed spatial constraints.

Then we compare the segmentation performance with and without the use of the distance features to the anatomical dense landmarks, and also the results with different number of classification iterations. The results in Fig. 3d demonstrate the effectiveness of the distance features to dense landmarks and iterative

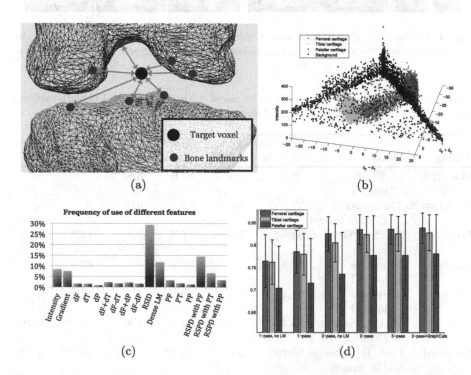

Fig. 3. (a) Distances to densely registered bone landmarks encode anatomical position of a voxel. (b) Feature scatter plot: intensity and distance features separate tibial cartilage from femoral and patellar cartilages. (c) Frequency of each feature selected by the classifier in the 2nd pass. (d) A comparison of segmentation performance (DSC): 1-pass/2-pass forests without using distance to landmark (LM) features; 1-pass/2-pass/3-pass forests using distance to landmark features; 2-pass forests with graph cuts optimization (3-fold cross validation).

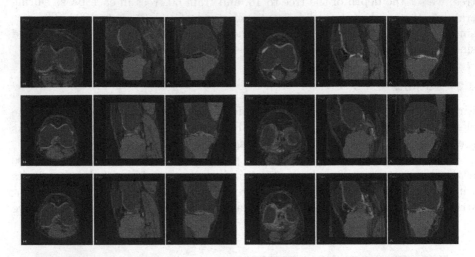

Fig. 4. Example bone segmentations. Each case has three views, from left to right: transversal plane, sagittal plane, coronal plane. Red: femur; green: tibia; blue: patella.

Table 2. Performance of our method compared with other state-of-the-art cartilage segmentation methods: mean DSC and standard deviation.

Author	Dataset	Fem. Cart. DSC Mean %	Std. %	Tib. Cart. DSC Mean %	Std. %	Pat. Cart. DSC Mean %	Std. %
Shan [23]	18 SPGR images	78.2	5.2	82.6	3.8	–	–
Folkesson [2]	139 Esaote C-Span images	77	8.0	81	6.0	–	–
Fripp [4]	20 FS SPGR images	84.8	7.6	82.6	8.3	83.3	13.5
Lee [6]	10 images in OAI	82.5	–	80.8	–	82.1	–
Yin [5]	60 images in OAI	84	4	80	4	80	4
	OAI, D_1 subset (58 images)	85.47	3.10	84.96	3.82	78.56	9.38
Proposed	OAI, D_2 subset (58 images)	85.20	3.65	83.52	4.08	80.79	7.40
method	OAI, D_3 subset (60 images)	84.22	3.05	82.74	3.84	78.12	9.63
	OAI, overall (176 images)	84.96	3.30	83.74	4.00	79.16	8.88

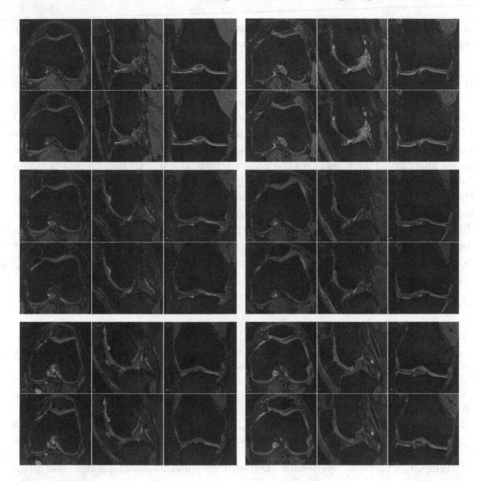

Fig. 5. Examples cartilage segmentations compared with ground truth. Each case has six images: segmentation results in upper row, ground truth in lower row. Red: femoral cartilage; green: tibial cartilage; blue: patellar cartilage.

classification with semantic context forests. In particular, 2-pass random forests achieve significant performance improvement, whereas the gain seems quite negligible by adding more passes.

Finally, the quantitative results (2-pass classification) are listed in Table 2 together with the numbers reported in the earlier literature. Because the datasets used are different by all these approaches, the numbers in the table are only for reference. Note that only our experiments are based on a relatively large dataset. As shown in the table, we achieved high performance with regard to the femoral and tibial cartilage, whereas the DSC of patellar cartilage is notably lower than the other two cartilages. This is partly because the size of patellar cartilage is much smaller than femoral and tibial cartilage, so that the same amount of segmentation error will result in lower DSC. Besides, some patellar cartilage annotations in the dataset do not appear very consistent with others. Example segmentation results are shown in Fig. 5.

5   Conclusion

We have presented a new approach to segment the three knee cartilages in 3-D MR images, which effectively exploits the semantic context information in the knee joint. By using the distance features to the bone surface as well as to the dense anatomical landmarks on the bone surface, the spatial constraints between cartilages and bones are incorporated without the need of explicit extraction of the bone cartilage interface. Furthermore, the use of multi-pass iterative classification with semantic context forests provides more spatial constraints between different cartilages to further improve the segmentation. The experiment validation shows the effectiveness of this method. Ongoing work include the joint bone-and-cartilage voxel classification in the iterative classification framework.

References

1. Graichen, H., Eisenhart-Rothe, R., Vogl, T., Englmeier, K.H., Eckstein, F.: Quantitative assessment of cartilage status in osteoarthritis by quantitative magnetic resonance imaging. Arthritis Rheumatism (2004)
2. Folkesson, J., Dam, E., Olsen, O., Pettersen, P., Christiansen, C.: Segmenting articular cartilage automatically using a voxel classification approach. IEEE Trans. Med. Imag. **26**(1), 106–115 (2007)
3. Vincent, G., Wolstenholme, C., Scott, I., Bowes, M.: Fully automatic segmentation of the knee joint using active appearance models. In: Medical Image Analysis for the Clinic: A Grand Challenge (2010)
4. Fripp, J., Crozier, S., Warfield, S., Ourselin, S.: Automatic segmentation and quantitative analysis of the articular cartilages from magnetic resonance images of the knee. IEEE Trans. Med. Imag. **29**(1), 55–64 (2010)
5. Yin, Y., Zhang, X., Williams, R., Wu, X., Anderson, D., Sonka, M.: Logismos - layered optimal graph image segmentation of multiple objects and surfaces: cartilage segmentation in the knee joint. IEEE Trans. Med. Imag. **29**(12), 2023–2037 (2010)
6. Lee, S., Park, S.H., Shim, H., Yun, I.D., Lee, S.U.: Optimization of local shape and appearance probabilities for segmentation of knee cartilage in 3-d mr images. CVIU **115**(12), 1710–1720 (2011)
7. Li, K., Wu, X., Chen, D., Sonka, M.: Optimal surface segmentation in volumetric images-a graph-theoretic approach. IEEE Trans. PAMI **28**(1), 119–134 (2006)
8. Tu, Z., Bai, X.: Auto-context and its application to high-level vision tasks and 3d brain image segmentation. IEEE Trans. PAMI **32**, 1744–1757 (2010)
9. Montillo, A., Shotton, J., Winn, J., Iglesias, J.E., Metaxas, D., Criminisi, A.: Entangled decision forests and their application for semantic segmentation of CT images. In: Székely, G., Hahn, H.K. (eds.) IPMI 2011. LNCS, vol. 6801, pp. 184–196. Springer, Heidelberg (2011)
10. Ling, H., Zheng, Y., Georgescu, B., Zhou, S.K., Suehling, M.: Hierarchical learning-based automatic liver segmentation. In: CVPR (2008)

11. Zheng, Y., Barbu, A., Georgescu, M., Scheuring, M., Comaniciu, D.: Four-chamber heart modeling and automatic segmentation for 3D cardiac CT volumes using marginal space learning and steerable features. IEEE Trans. Med. Imag. **27**(11), 1668–1681 (2008)
12. Myronenko, A., Song, X.: Point set registration: coherent point drift. IEEE Trans. PAMI **32**(12), 2262–2275 (2010)
13. Cootes, T., Taylor, C., Cooper, D., Graham, J.: Active shape models-their training and application. CVIU **61**(1), 38–59 (1995)
14. Grady, L.: Random walks for image segmentation. IEEE Trans. PAMI **28**(11), 1768–1783 (2006)
15. Shotton, J., Fitzgibbon, A., Cook, M., Sharp, T., Finocchio, M., Moore, R., Kipman, A., Blake, A.: Real-time human pose recognition in parts from single depth images. In: CVPR, pp. 1297–1304, June 2011
16. Lepetit, V., Lagger, P., Fua, P.: Randomized trees for real-time keypoint recognition. In: CVPR, vol. 2, pp. 775–781, June 2005
17. Quinlan, J.R.: Induction of decision trees. Mach. Learn. **1**(1), 81–106 (1986)
18. Breiman, L.: Random forests. Mach. Learn. **45**(1), 5–32 (2001)
19. Wang, Q., Ou, Y., Julius, A.A., Boyer, K.L., Kim, M.J.: Tracking *tetrahymena pyriformis* cells using decision trees. In: ICPR, November 2012
20. Zikic, D., Glocker, B., Konukoglu, E., Shotton, J., Criminisi, A., Ye, D., Demiralp, C., Thomas, O., Das, T., Jena, R., et al.: Context-sensitive classification forests for segmentation of brain tumor tissues. In: MICCAI (2012)
21. Boykov, Y., Veksler, O., Zabih, R.: Fast approximate energy minimization via graph cuts. IEEE Trans. PAMI **23**(11), 1222–1239 (2001)
22. Boykov, Y., Funka-Lea, G.: Graph cuts and efficient n-d image segmentation. Int. J. Comput. Vis. **70**(2), 109–131 (2006)
23. Shan, L., Charles, C., Niethammer, M.: Automatic atlas-based three-label cartilage segmentation from mr knee images. In: 2012 IEEE Workshop on Mathematical Methods in Biomedical Image Analysis, pp. 241–246, January 2012

Detection and Localization

Local Phase-Based Fast Ray Features for Automatic Left Ventricle Apical View Detection in 3D Echocardiography

João S. Domingos[1](✉), Eduardo Lima[2], Paul Leeson[2], and J. Alison Noble[1]

[1] Department of Engineering Science, University of Oxford, Oxford, UK
[2] Department of Cardiovascular Medicine, John Radcliffe Hospital, Oxford, UK
domingos.domingos@eng.ox.ar.uk

Abstract. 3D echocardiography is an imaging modality that enables a more complete and rapid cardiac function assessment. However, as a time-consuming procedure, it calls upon automatic view detection to enable fast 3D volume navigation and analysis. We propose a combinatorial model- and machine learning-based left ventricle (LV) apical view detection method consisting of three steps: first, multiscale local phase-based 3D boundary detection is used to fit a deformable model to the boundaries of the LV blood pool. After candidate slice extraction around the derived mid axis of the LV segmentation, we propose the use of local phase-based Fast Ray features to complement conventional Haar features in an AdaBoost-based framework for automated standardized LV apical view detection. Evaluation performed on a combination of healthy volunteers and clinical patients with different image quality and ultrasound probes show that apical plane views can be accurately identified in a 360 degree swipe of 3D frames.

1 Introduction

3D echocardiography (3DE) is a cardiac imaging modality intended to replace common 2D echocardiography in clinical practice. Several research studies [1,2] have demonstrated that 3DE improves upon multi-chamber volumetric analysis, providing more precise information about its pathophysiology. However, interpretation and quantitative analysis of 3D echocardiographic data is time consuming, limiting its use in routine clinical practice. Therefore, detection of standardized planes in 3DE is of crucial importance to automate clinical workflow.

Recently, machine learning classification approaches have been proposed to address this challenge in rest 3DE. In [3], the authors proposed automatic 3D detection of standardized planes by using a database-driven knowledge-based approach to build an automated supervised learning framework. The method extracts Haar-like and steerable features from each standard view and creates a probabilistic model which is then used to search for planes in the hypothesis space. In [2], the authors presented an automatic approach for alignment of standard apical and short-axis views in 3D echocardiography, correcting them

B. Menze et al. (Eds.): MCV 2013, LNCS 8331, pp. 119–129, 2014.
DOI: 10.1007/978-3-319-05530-5_12, © Springer International Publishing Switzerland 2014

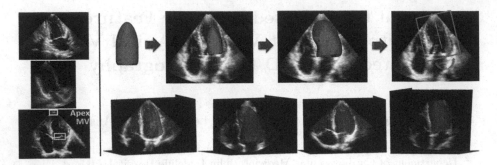

Fig. 1. Standard apical views of the heart (*left column*): A2C (*top*), A3C and A4C (*bottom*). In order to obtain meaningful 2D candidate views, a LV deformable model is automatically placed in the LV heart chamber and iteratively fitted to the endocardium edges until deformation displacement is minimal (*right column, top row*). The principal component of this surface is then extracted and a 360° swipe of the 3D volume is performed around the LV centerline, yielding 360 candidate slices for classification. 3D LV blood pool segmentation and respective centerline examples are shown above (*right column, bottom row*). On the bottom of the *left column*, MV in light blue represents the two insertions of the mitral valve and apex in yellow the apex of the heart.

for out-of-plane motion. In [4], the authors proposed a database guided detection of anatomical landmark points in 3D echocardiography for Haar feature-based automatic extraction of standard views using a small database with artificial variations. In [5], the authors proposed a real time Haar feature-based boosting framework to automatically detect apical standard views over the full extent of a given 3D frame. In [6], the authors propose a one-step approach for standard view extraction from a 3D volume using a class-specific regression random forest voting framework validated on a limited dataset. These techniques commonly focus on intensity-based feature detection and, in some cases, rely on the geometrical constraints between anatomically standard views (A2C to A3C: 30°–40° and A2C to A4C: 90°) in order to correctly detect them. However, in ultrasound images the feature detection task is very challenging due to speckle, poor signal-to-noise-ratio and low-contrast nature of the images and thus the previous intensity based methods tend not to perform very well when applied to echocardiograms of both healthy volunteers and clinical patients, different ultrasound probes, and different acquisition-dependent dataset quality.

The motivation behind this work is the task of detecting the three most common apical views of the LV (Left Ventricle): A2C, A3C and A4C (Apical 2, 3 and 4 Chamber) views depicted in Fig. 1. As in [5], we propose an Adaboost-based standard view detectors that fully scan 2D slices, derived from a precomputed 3D LV segmentation, searching for a combination of a small number of anatomical landmark points that strongly represent and identify each one of these views. Because Haar features are inefficient in the task of detecting highly deformable objects such as heart chambers, valves and walls, a comprehensive training set would have to be provided with a full range of object deformations, including the large deviations that usually require weaker learners. To overcome these limitations and improve feature detection robustness, we explore efficient Fast Ray features [7], or Rays, based on local phase information retrieved by the Feature Asymmetry (FA) measure. In addition to the Rays advantages, it has been shown previously that ultrasound images respond well to this local phase based technique due to its reduced sensitivity to speckle and intensity invariance [8].

2 Methods

2.1 LV Blood Pool Segmentation

With 3D volume slicing in mind, a deformable LV anatomical model of the LV endocardium was initially used to segment the LV blood pool of 3D echocardiograms at end-diastole. Similar to [9], the Doo-Sabin subdivision scheme [10] was the method used for generalising binary refinement of biquadratic B-splines to a non-rectangular control mesh. This subdivision surface is automatically initialized via circular Hough transform accumulation maps obtained from each volume transverse plane (short axis view) and is entirely represented by 24 control vertices which only locally deform the end surface composed of 9600 surface points, depicted in Fig. 1. 3D blood pool boundary detection is performed iteratively by probing 3D FA maps derived from the monogenic signal and detecting step-like edges, i.e. blood pool or endocardium border. In contrast to the similar surface implemented in [5,9], we rely on an iterative surface deformation process that deforms to 3D multiscale local phase FA measurements instead of uni dimensional ones.

2.2 Monogenic Signal and Edge Measurements

Local phase encodes local structural information and can be obtained by convolving a 1D signal with a pair of band pass quadrature filters. Common filter choices are the isotropic log-Gabor, $G^{lg}(\omega = exp(-\frac{log(\omega/\omega_0)^2}{2log^2(\kappa_{\omega 0})}))$, and Gaussian-derivative, $G^{gd}(\omega) = \omega.exp(-\omega^2\sigma^2)$, filters where κ is related to the bandwidth of the filter, ω_0 is the centre frequency of the filter and σ is the isotropic spread of the filter. The value $0 < \kappa_{\omega 0} < 1$ ensures a constant shape-bandwidth ratio over scales.

Originally derived from the phase congruency measure, the FA measure has proven to be a contrast-invariant measure of symmetry and less sensitive to ultrasound speckle [8]. It was recently modified in [8] using a high dimensional generalization of the analytic signal, the monogenic signal [11], being based on the Riesz transform which is used instead of the Hilbert transform. The spatial representations of these filters are of the form: $h_1(x,y) = -x/(2\pi(x^2 + y^2)^3/2))$ and $h_2(x,y) = -y/(2\pi(x^2 + y^2)^3/2))$. In practice, the image is first convolved with an even isotropic band-pass filter $bf(x,y)$ yielding the even component of the monogenic signal: $even(x,y) = I_b f(x,y) = bf(x,y) * I(x,y)$. Thereafter, the band-passed image $I_b f(x,y)$ is filtered with the Riesz filter to produce the odd (anti-symmetric) components: $odd_1(x,y) = h_1(x,y) * Ibf(x,y)$ and $odd_2(x,y) = h_2(x,y) * Ibf(x,y)$. Finally, the local phase $\varphi(x,y)$ of image $I(x,y)$ is defined as $\varphi(x,y) = arctan(even(x,y)/odd(x,y))$ and the monogenic signal $I_M(x,y)$ is expressed in the following form [11]:

$$I_M(x,y) = [I_bf(x,y), h_1(x,y) * I_bf(x,y), h_2(x,y) * I_bf(x,y)] \qquad (1)$$

3D Multiscale local phase image maps were then computed by averaging the local phase computed at 3 scales of filter wavelength of $[30, 36, 42]$ pixels and $[4, 7, 10]$ pixels for the $G^{lg}(\omega)$ and $G^{gd}(\omega)$ filters respectively. Although the $G^{gd}(\omega)$ filter provides a much cleaner boundary localization and no ringing artifacts [8], stronger boundary values are provided by the $G^{lg}(\omega)$ filter which are necessary to distinguish between endocardium border and, for example, trabeculation boundary. The remaining filter parameters were set up as reported in [8] and the resulting filter bank was found to give acceptable results. The 3D multiscale FA measure map for each 3D image can then be determined by:

$$FA_{3D}(x,y) = \sum_s \frac{\lfloor [|odd_s(x,y)| - |even_s(x,y)|] - T_s \rfloor}{\sqrt{(even_s(x,y)^2 + odd_s(x,y)^2)} + \epsilon} \qquad (2)$$

where $\lfloor . \rfloor$ denotes zeroing of any negative values, s traverses of a range of scales, factor $T_s = exp(mean(log(\sqrt{(even_s(x,y)^2 + odd_s(x,y)^2)})))$ is a noise compensation term representing the maximum response that could be generated from noise alone in the signal and ϵ is a small constant to prevent division by zero.

In order to detect the 3D LV endocardium wall, we compute 3D multiscale local phase, FA, and gradient component maps (each 3D echocardiogram takes $\sim$10 s to compute using Matlab and 8 cores of an Intel Xeon X5660 computer). The local phase and FA maps are individually thresholded at 0.3 to enhance the LV and RV (Right Ventricle) myocardium edges. After summing both the individual maps obtained from each filter, $G^{lg}(\omega)$ and $G^{gd}(\omega)$, the resulting FA map is again thresholded at 0.2 for the same reason. Blood pool border search is performed on a set of 384 sampling lines, normal to the deformable surface, by sampling and probing the previously obtained 3D volume maps along these vectors. At each of these normals, we use the FA measure to iteratively find and evaluate possible endocardial edges, after which the blood pool surface is deformed according to the estimated displacement. This process is repeated until the global deformation displacement between iterations is insignificant. Thus, LV global shape information plays an important part in the deformable surface evolution, which in turn makes use of the known good response of ultrasound images to the local phase based FA measure.

2.3   3D Volume Slicing: LV Long Axis Determination

Singular value decomposition is performed on the mean-centered data of the 9600 deformable surface points to extract the LV first principal component, i.e. the long axis fit to the LV blood pool. Slicing finally occurs by rotation of a plane over the found axis in a 360° swipe of the 3D frame. Note that the estimation of the LV mid line is of the utmost importance to the alignment of the LV upon volume slicing since it allows all candidate slices to be aligned with the heart apex and MVC (Mitral Valve Centre), therefore strengthening anatomical landmark locations and improving the knowledge on the position of chambers and walls (edges) on the slices. In comparison with [5], our long axis determination method does not require any time-consuming automatic centerline tracing computation and thus runs quickly.

2.4 Haar and Ray Feature Sets

Low-level but powerful features derived from the Haar wavelets were used since they have proved to effectively encode the domain knowledge, in the form of locally oriented intensity differences [4]. Haar features are attractive for their use of efficient integral images and hence were extracted in a sliding window fashion in the form of seven different types of rectangle features depicted in Fig. 2. Haars are sensitive to edges and lines which greatly benefit the detection of features of endocardium walls and heart chambers. Nevertheless, they depend on reliable cues defined at precise locations, resulting in a need for additional weak learners to represent large deviations in the training set.

To efficiently and robustly recognise deformable or irregular shapes, such as heart cavities, we take advantage of the complementary information provided by Fast Ray features [7]. These are comprised of four adaptations of the function $\mathbf{c} = c(\mathbf{I}, \mathbf{m}, \theta)$, which outputs the location $\mathbf{c}$ of the nearest contour pixel in image $\mathbf{I}$ to the location $\mathbf{m}$ in the direction of angle θ. As depicted in Fig. 2, Rays can

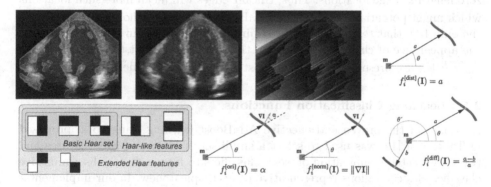

Fig. 2. The feature pool comprises 2-, 3- and 4-rectangle combinations of Haars for a minimum filter size of 26 with a step size of 4 for 85×108 slices (*bottom, right*); and four types of Rays (*schematic images* adapted from [7]). As an example, computation of $f_i^{[dist]}$ features starts with slicing of 3D multiscale FA maps (*in green, top row*) and 2D thinning of the resulting edge maps (*in red, top row*). The resulting Ray distance feature map for $\theta = 30°$ and its schematic representation are shown in the (*top row, right*). In the former, dark and bright intensities correspond to short and long distances respectively.

be computed by recalling the gradient at the last contour the scan line crossed. The Ray feature set is defined as follows [7]:

Distance and Distance Difference Features. While the distance feature, $f_i^{[dist]}(\mathbf{m}_i) = \| c(\mathbf{I}, \mathbf{m}_i, \theta_i) - \mathbf{m}_i \|$, computes the absolute distance to the closest edge point in a given direction, the dominant and scale invariant distance difference feature, $f_i^{[diff]}(\mathbf{m}_i) = \frac{\|c(\mathbf{I},\mathbf{m}_i,\theta_i)-\mathbf{m}_i\|-\|c(\mathbf{I},\mathbf{m}_i,\theta_i')-\mathbf{m}_i\|}{\|c(\mathbf{I},\mathbf{m}_i,\theta_i)-\mathbf{m}_i\|}$, compares the relative distances from a given image $\mathbf{m}_i$ location to the nearest boundaries in two search directions with angles θ_i and θ_i'.

Orientation Feature. The orientation feature characterizes objects by their contour orientation and computes the orientation of the nearest boundary in direction θ as $f_i^{[ori]}(\mathbf{m}_i) = \frac{\nabla I(c(\mathbf{I},\mathbf{m}_i,\theta_i))}{\|\nabla I(c(\mathbf{I},\mathbf{m}_i,\theta_i))\|} \cdot (cos\theta_i, sin\theta_i)^\top$, where $\nabla I(c)$ is the gradient of image $\mathbf{I}$ at $\mathbf{c}$.

Norm Feature. The norm feature, $f_i^{[norm]}(\mathbf{m}_i) = \| \nabla I(c(\mathbf{I}, \mathbf{m}_i, \theta_i)) \|$, computes the gradient strength of the nearest contour in direction θ.

Since Rays depend on meaningful edges and instead of using standard filtering techniques that do not respond well to ultrasound images, we extracted thinned binary edge masks $\mathbf{B}$ and gradient approximations ∇I from the precomputed 3D multiscale local phase maps. Ray extraction was performed at every second pixel location in the scan window, with a 30° angular interval and $f_i^{[diff]}$ angle pairs set as a unique combination of these angles.

Note that although edges in $\mathbf{B}$ are not required to be thinned, Rays will have zero length at edge locations. Thus, thicker edges will mean more such locations which might potentially confuse the AdaBoost learning method. Since $f_i^{[norm]}$ is the only Ray that tests intensity in $\mathbf{B}$ and is therefore useful for characterizing the appearance of chamber contours of the heart, we expect to witness a lower $f_i^{[norm]}$ feature presence in the AdaBoost final strong classifier.

2.5   Learning Classification Functions

A variant of the proven and effective AdaBoost learning framework, proposed in Table 1 of [12] was used to select a small set of Haar and Ray features and train a weighted combination of weak classifiers to form a strong discriminative classifier of local regions representative of each apical view. In our implementation, these weak classifiers were based on the difference of the cumulative sum of the positive (apical LV standard view) and negative (non-apical LV standard view) weighted histograms. The overall method involves a first step of feature extraction, followed by training of weak classifiers, $h_j(x)$, and finally, automatic feature selection with high relevance. The final strong classifier is defined as:

$$h(x) = \begin{cases} 1 & \sum_{t=1}^{T} \alpha_t h_t(x) \geq \frac{1}{2} \sum_{t=1}^{T} \alpha_t \\ 0 & \text{otherwise} \end{cases} \tag{3}$$

where the strong classifier threshold, $\frac{1}{2}\sum_{t=1}^{T}\alpha_t$, is designed to yield a low error rate on the training data. A lower threshold will produce a higher detection rate and a higher false positive rate and vice versa.

3   Experimental Results

3.1   3D Echocardiogram Database

The implemented plane detectors were tested on a dataset of 30 healthy volunteers and 36 clinical patients with suspected valve disease and coronary heart disease. Echocardiograms were recorded using a Philips iE33 xMATRIX Echocardiography System (X3-1 and X5-1 probes). After 3D echocardiogram slicing, each set of 360 candidate slices was annotated for A2C, A3C and A4C standard view intervals, i.e. a given apical view is considered to be present in a continuous range of angles that are very similar in their content and thus represent the same best apical standard view. The annotated intervals range from 6 to 32 slices.

3.2   Validation Methodology

In order to validate the LV long axis centerlines obtained by principal component analysis of the deformable surface points, manual iterative 3D LV landmark annotation of the heart apex and MVC, depicted in Fig. 1, was performed by an expert cardiologist according to the same protocol described in Fig. 1 in [4]. Although the data used in these studies is not the same to help place this work in perspective, a comparison of the validation results with current literature is made in Table 1(a). 3D LV blood pool segmentation and centerline extraction take ∼13 s (mean time) to compute using Python and VTK on a single core of an Intel Core i7-870 computer with 8GB RAM, but can be calculated in real time as demonstrated in [2].

   Our experiment results, depicted in Table 1(b), compare the classification performance of Haar and Ray features for three classification functions implemented to detect each apical view from the 360 candidate slices. In addition a comparison is made between classifiers based on Haar only (H), Rays only (R), and both $(H + R)$. Initially we fixed the AdaBoost number of iterations, T, each of which form a weak learner. This parameter was empirically selected based on ROC (Receiver Operating Characteristic) curves for each of the feature sets. We mainly demonstrate results for the A4C plane detector, since this is the view with the biggest structural difference (four easily differentiable heart chambers) to the other views and non-standard view slices, and therefore is the detector expected to have the best performance. The remaining apical standard views can then be easily derived from the A4C ones using their known geometrical relationships. In the final experiment we test unseen data sequences of 360 slices and show how accurate the proposed framework is by performing 3-fold cross validation of results with the dataset (66×360 slices) split into training and testing cases. The negative training set contained every sixth (minimum annotated

Table 1. (a) Comparison of landmark detection errors with current literature (Mitral Valve Centre, MVC). (b) Area under the ROC curves (AUC) for each plane detector, for $T_{H_1} = 100$, $T_{H_2} = 200$, $T_{R_1} = 300$ and $T_{R_2} = 500$ Adaboost iterations (*top table*). AxC view detection performance (Accuracy, *Acc*) of feature sets, where H, R and $H+R$ are Haars, Rays and the combination of both respectively, for the best performing T of $200H + 500R$ (*bottom table*). $L - dev$ and $R - dev$ are the mean slice distances (in slices) between the ground truth interval limits and the detected interval limits (Left- and Right- side, respectively) regarding the $H + R$ detector.

(a) LV landmark detection errors

	Apex (mm)	MVC (mm)
Our method	7.1 ±5.7	7.2 ±5.3
Karavides [4]	7.5 ±3.3	5.0 ±2.5
Orderud [2]	8.4 ±3.5	3.6 ±1.8
Lu [3]	4.5 ±3.5	3.6 ±3.1
Leung [13]	7.6 ±4.8	4.5 ±2.9
Van Stralen [14]	14.7 ±8.6	8.4 ±5.7
Interobserver [13]	7.1 ±2.9	3.8 ±1.3
Intraobserver [13]	5.2 ±2.0	3.3 ±1.5

(b) AxC view classification results

AxC View	H_1 AUC	H_2 AUC	R_1 AUC	R_2 AUC
A2C vs All	0.812	0.824	0.777	0.796
A3C vs All	0.902	0.896	0.861	0.895
A4C vs All	0.904	0.926	0.896	0.911

AxC View	H Acc (%)	R Acc (%)	H+R Acc (%)	L-dev (slices)	R-dev (slices)
A2C vs All	36.4	29.5	51.5	11.5 ±8.1	11.8 ±9.6
A3C vs All	72.7	65.9	77.3	9.0 ±6.4	11.9 ±10.1
A4C vs All	66.7	53.0	90.9	6.9 ±4.1	11.0 ±8.8

interval) non-apical view slice, as opposed to the positive training set where all AxC view slices annotated by the expert were included.

Apical view detection was considered successful when there was more than one annotated slice inside the detected AxC (A2C, A3C or A4C) view interval as depicted in red in Fig. 3. Table 1(b) bottom shows the detection results. $H + R$ feature precomputation ($\sim$50 s) and single AxC view detection on the 360 candidate slices ($\sim$0.12 s) takes a total of $\sim$50 s using Matlab and 8 cores of an Intel Xeon X5660 computer with 48 GB RAM.

3.3   Discussion of Proposed Model- and AdaBoost-Based Method

Generally, comparing the LV long axis validation results, represented in Table 1(a), with the ones given by current literature we find a similar detection error for the apex centre and a slightly higher error for the MVC. Note that in [13], although results are better, the method registers landmarks in stress images based on the landmarks in rest images which makes the detection job easier. Regarding the method in [3], the much larger database (244 training datasets from 326 patients) may explain why they achieve such a good performance. Finally, we had our dataset manually annotated only once by one expert and therefore we have no measure of the interobserver and intraobserver variabilities and hence ground truth error estimate. This fact is significant to both the LV centerline and plane detectors validation. Nevertheless, in the former case we are still able to achieve a very similar detection error to the interobserver variation in [13] for the apex landmark.

After training the three plane detectors, we analyzed ROC curves and AUCs in order to gain a first impression of the classifiers performance, represented in Table 1(b). As expected, the A4C view detector outperforms the others due to

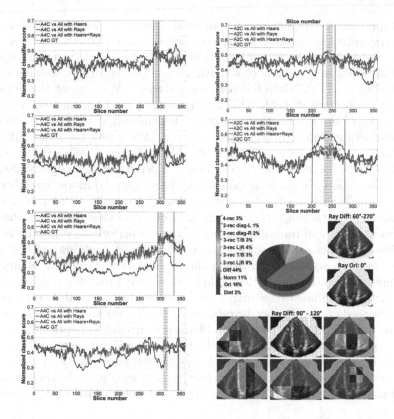

Fig. 3. Examples of A4C (*left column*) and A2C (*top right corner*) normalized detector scores and apical standard view interval detection (in red) for all slices in six different test volumes. The test volume on the (*bottom right corner*) is an example of a misdetection by the A4C detector. The dotted line marks the strong Adaboost threshold formalized in Eq. 3. The pie chart depicts the A4C AdaBoost feature preferences. Examples of highly scored features selected during training of the AdaBoost A4C $H + R$ detector are represented below (*bottom right corner*). Due to the 3D slicing procedure, candidate slices vary in size and hence a global binary mask, depicted as the point pattern envolving the echocardiogram 'cones', had to be created to include all of those.

its rich structural information (higher number of heart cavities than any other slice). A higher AUC yields a better apical view detector outputting fewer false positives, and vice versa. ROC analysis also demonstrated that in the context of apical view finding by extensive search of 2D slices, $T = {\sim}20$ Haar-based weak classifiers and $T = {\sim}50$ Ray-based ones are enough to reach a significant AUC measure in all detectors, point from which AUC increases very little with the increase of T. Nevertheless, and because at run time we simply evaluate a specific number of weak learners in the whole slice, we choose a significantly higher number of weak learners for each feature type: $T = 200$ for Haars and $T = 500$ for Rays. From this point on, there was no improvement in the AUC.

More importantly, a higher number of weak learners is also required since it demonstrated to improve the precision (a decrease in the $L - dev$ and $R - dev$ number of slices reported in Table 1(b)) of all detected apical view intervals.

Apical view detection was considered successful when there was more than one GT slice inside the detected AxC view interval. We present the detection results in the bottom of Table 1(b). Unsurprisingly, the implemented A4C view detector outperforms the other detectors demonstrating that the poorer the structural information is, in a given apical view (A2C case), the more difficult it is for AdaBoost to pick up weak learners able to detect it. With the exception of the A4C detector, both the $L - dev$ and $R - dev$ results are slightly high and may require a more robust solution such as a cascaded AdaBoost classifier.

Results in Table 1(b) also demonstrate that although Fast Ray features cannot replace and outperform Haars in the task of apical view detection, they can complement them and improve the final detection performance just by considering distances from arbitrary locations to the nearest contours. Although the proposed local phase-based FA method allows generation of different binary edge maps depending on the chosen threshold level, we only presented results for Rays precalculated on thinned edge maps. Hence, an evaluation of different FA map thresholds needs to be further investigated. Finally, we also demonstrate that AdaBoost prefers Rays features for problems with irregular shapes such as heart cavities, since amongst the Rays with the highest AdaBoost scores, α, the corresponding image positions are almost always located near the RV. This happens because this chamber appears and disappears constantly with the rotation of the moving plane over the LV mid axis, making it a structure with a highly irregular shape.

4   Conclusion

We have developed an improved fully automated combinatorial model- and machine learning-based framework to detect LV A4C standard views in healthy and clinical 3D echocardiograms of different image qualities. The remaining A2C and A3C views can be extracted from the A4C view using the known geometrical relationships between apical standard views. We demonstrated that Fast Ray features complement Rays and improve the detector performance when compared to a Haar-based detector. A2C and A3C view detection still remains a challenging task that needs further research. One limitation of the proposed method is the requirement of an accurate LV mid-axis extraction method, since the plane detectors will only retrieve local information from 2D slices obtained from a plane rotation on this centerline. Therefore, the proposed method needs to be tested on a larger training set in the future to assess this.

Acknowledgments. The authors are grateful for the financial support provided by the RCUK Centre for Doctoral Training in Healthcare Innovation (EP/G036861/1) and EPSRC grant EP/G030693/1. We would also like to thank Richard Stebbing, Kevin Smith, Carlos Arteta and Mohammad Yaqub for the helpful discussions and advice.

References

1. Mor-Avi, V., Sugeng, L., Lang, R.: Real-time 3-dimensional echocardiography: an integral component of the routine echocardiographic examination in adult patients? Circulation **119**(2), 314 (2009)
2. Orderud, F., Torp, H., Rabben, S.: Automatic alignment of standard views in 3d echocardiograms using real-time tracking. In: Proceedings of SPIE Ultrasonic Imaging and Signal Processing, vol. 7265, pp. 1–7. (2009)
3. Lu, X., Georgescu, B., Zheng, Y., Otsuki, J., Comaniciu, D.: Automated detection of planes from three-dimensional echocardiographic data. US Patent App. 12/186,815, 6 August 2008
4. Karavides, T., Leung, K., Paclik, P., Hendriks, E., Bosch, J.: Database guided detection of anatomical landmark points in 3d images of the heart. In: IEEE International Symposium on Biomedical Imaging: From Nano to Macro, pp. 1089–1092. IEEE (2010)
5. Domingos, J., Augustine, D., Leeson, P., Noble, J.: Automatic left ventricle apical plane detection in 3d echocardiography. In: Proceedings of SPIE Medical Imaging (2013)
6. Chykeyuk, K., Yaqub, M., Noble, J.: Class-specific regression random forest for accurate extraction of standard planes from 3d echocardiography. In: MICCAI International Workshop on Machine Learning in Medical Imaging (2013)
7. Smith, K., Carleton, A., Lepetit, V.: Fast ray features for learning irregular shapes. In: IEEE 12th International Conference on Computer Vision, pp. 397–404. IEEE (2009)
8. Rajpoot, K., Grau, V., Noble, J.: Local-phase based 3d boundary detection using monogenic signal and its application to real-time 3-d echocardiography images. In: IEEE International Symposium on Biomedical Imaging: From Nano to Macro. ISBI'09, pp. 783–786. IEEE (2009)
9. Orderud, F., Rabben, S.: Real-time 3d segmentation of the left ventricle using deformable subdivision surfaces. In: IEEE Conference on Computer Vision and Pattern Recognition. CVPR 2008, pp. 1–8. IEEE (2008)
10. Doo, D., Sabin, M.: Behaviour of recursive division surfaces near extraordinary points. Comput. Aided Des. **10**, 356–360 (1978)
11. Felsberg, M., Sommer, G.: The monogenic signal. IEEE Trans. Signal Process. **49**, 3136–3144 (2001)
12. Viola, P., Jones, M.: Robust real-time face detection. Int. J. Comput. Vis. **57**, 137–154 (2004)
13. Esther Leung, K., van Stralen, M., Nemes, A., Voormolen, M., van Burken, G.,Geleijnse, M., Ten Cate, F., Reiber, J., de Jong, N., van der Steen, A., et al.: Sparse registration for three-dimensional stress echocardiography. IEEE Trans. Med. Imag. **27**, 1568–1579 (2008)
14. Van Stralen, M., Leung, K., Voormolen, M., De Jong, N., Van der Steen, A., Reiber, J., Bosch, J.: Time continuous detection of the left ventricular long axis and the mitral valve plane in 3-d echocardiography. Ultrasound Med. Biol. **34**, 196–207 (2008)

Automatic Aorta Detection
in Non-contrast 3D Cardiac CT Images
Using Bayesian Tracking Method

Mingna Zheng[1,2]($\boxtimes$), J. Jeffery Carr[2], and Yaorong Ge[1,2,3]

[1] Virginia Tech-Wake Forest University School
of Biomedical Engineering and Sciences, Blacksburg, USA
[2] Wake Forest University School of Medicine, Winston-Salem, USA
[3] University of North Carolina Charlotte, Charlotte, USA
mzheng@wakehealth.edu

Abstract. Automatic aorta detection is important for the diagnosis and treatment planning of aortic diseases, such as acute aortic dissection and aneurysm. Manually labeling and tracking the aorta in a large amount of non-contrast CT images are time-consuming and labor-intensive. In this paper, we describe a fully automated method to tackle this problem. We apply General Hough Transom(GHT) to detect the approximately circular shape of the aorta on 2D slices. The k-means clustering algorithm is used to identify two initial points for subsequent vessel tracking. In order to correctly detect the centerline of aorta, the proposed method based on the Bayesian estimation framework incorporates aorta-related prior knowledge. Our approach can handle the variations in the radius along the tubular vessel and the morphological differences of the aortic arch. Initial results on 24 CT datasets from a longitudinal cardiovascular study are encouraging.

1 Introduction

Aortic dissection is the most common incidence of the aorta, and it is a medical emergency and can quickly lead to death. The diagnosis is made with medical imaging modalities, such as CT and Magnetic Resonance(MR) imaging. Whereas conventional angiography has been the standard for arterial imaging, computed tomographic angiography(CTA) has been used with increasing frequency as an alternative to the more invasive conventional angiography [8]. For assessment of aorta in the cardiac CT images, an expert has to segment the aorta slice by slice using a pointing tool. This task can be tedious and time consuming, even for trained professionals. Additionally, the result highly depends on the user and has limited reproducibility. Therefore, a quick and accurate automated aorta detection system would be of great help.

1.1 The Structure of Aorta

The whole aorta is made of three parts: ascending aorta, descending aorta and aortic arch (Fig. 1). The ascending aorta extends upward from the aortic root

B. Menze et al. (Eds.): MCV 2013, LNCS 8331, pp. 130–137, 2014.
DOI: 10.1007/978-3-319-05530-5_13, © Springer International Publishing Switzerland 2014

to the place where the aorta begins to form an arch. The arch is the curved portion at the top of the aorta. The descending aorta begins from the arch and bends down into the body. The ascending and descending aorta are approximately straight tubular-shaped vessels in 3D view, but the aortic arch could have different distortions as shown in Fig. 2.

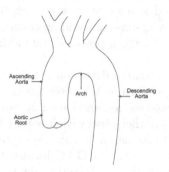

Fig. 1. The structure of the aorta.

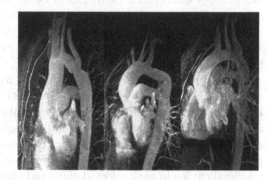

Fig. 2. Three different morphologies of the aortic arch after a coarctation repair [9].

1.2   Related Work

Since the aorta is a tubular structure, many generic tubular structure/vessel tracking methods have been applied to detect and segment it. Among the numerous vessel tracking methods in the literature, statistical vessel tracking methods have received considerable attention because they can incorporate prior knowledge into predicting the next possible location. Statistical tracking methods are centerline-based approaches, assuming the existence of a well-defined centerline. Because vessels are elongated structures of varying radii and curvatures, these algorithms search iteratively by estimating vessel parameters such as centerline point location and radius. Particle filtering, also known as the sequential Monte Carlo method, is recursive tracking scheme which can be used to estimate the Bayesian posterior distribution function (pdf) of a dynamic process with a set of discrete states. Particle filtering was first applied to vessel segmentation by Florin et al. [4]. In this research, the likelihood estimation relies on a Gaussian mixture model, which describes the intensity distribution of both vessels and hyper-intense areas caused by calcifications and stent. In Schaap et al. [10] study, vessel-related prior knowledge including information about radius changes, direction changes and intensity changes is integrated in to the Bayesian estimation framework. And in Lesage et al. study [7], a sampling scheme is proposed to reduce the number of samples to track the vessels.

Besides the above generic vessel tracking methods, there are some automated aorta segmentation algorithms proposed in the literature to detect and segment aorta in 3D images. Isgum et al. [6] proposed an atlas-based segmentation app-roach based on the combination of multiple registrations with focus on the ascending and descending aorta. Zhao et al. [11] described a semi-automatic method to segment aorta in MR images by manually selecting a seed point to initialize the fast march method. Biesdorf et al. [2] introduced a new joint segmentation and registration approach for the quantification of the aortic arch morphology that combines 3D model-based segmentation with elastic image reg-istration. Zheng et al. [12] presented a part-based segmentation approach that handles the whole aorta structure including the ascending, descending aorta and aortic arch. None of the previous work has ever adopted a probabilistic method for aorta detection.

In this paper, we present a novel method for automated detection of the whole aorta in the 3D cardiac CT images. Our method is based on the observation that the aortic lumen has an approximately circular cross section and therefore can be found with a proper circle detection technique. Another observation is that the aortic arch part has a strong bending that connects the ascending and descending parts together. First, we use the General Hough Transform (GHT) to localize two maximal circles in each selected slice, and then use k-means clustering algorithm to exclude the false results from the previous GHT step, and pick two initial points in the ascending and descending aorta respectively. Bayesian tracking framework is applied to track the vessel both upward and downward until it stops when no aortic region is detected or it reaches the volume border. The aorta-related prior knowledge that used for Bayesian tracking method includes the information about radius changes, direction changes, intensity changes and the spatial relationship changes between the ascending and descending aorta.

2   Methods

Our goal is to automatically detect and track the whole aorta in the 3D cardiac CT images. Figure 3 shows the outline of the proposed method. The automatic aorta detection proceeds by first selecting the initial points for vessel tracking. We use the circle GHT to detect the ascending and descending aorta in the 2D slices based on the assumption that the aortic lumen is circle-shaped in the cross-section view. Then we apply the k-means clustering method in 3D to exclude false results that generated from the previous GHT step, and select two initial points in both ascending and descending aorta. Initial points are not required to be in any specific location along the aorta, for example the aortic root or heart chamber, which are considered as good places to start 'bottom-up' or 'up-bottom' tracking in the previous works. Taking advantage of some aorta-related prior knowledge, the Bayesian tracking method is used to track both upward and downward in the 3D volumes. In addition, the preprocessing step that selects a range of interested CT slices by hand before the automated procedure is optional. The last step is to predict the approximate centerlines of missing or partially occluded aorta segments in order to keep the completeness of the whole centerline presentation.

The details of each step are described in the following subsections.

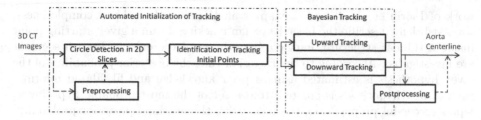

Fig. 3. The outline of the proposed automated detection method.

2.1 Preprocessing

Before the detection procedure starts, we may examine the input data volume and select only interested cardiac CT slices based on their DICOM information. This optional step minimizes the data volume to reduce memory requirements and execution time.

2.2 Automated Initialization of the Aorta Tracking

To start the segmentation, two seed points, one in the ascending and one in the descending aorta are required. Either the user selects these points manually, or they can be located automatically.

The automatic selection is divided into several phases. First, the approximate region of the heart is detected by calculating the average intensity of all axial slices. Starting from the slice with the highest average intensity, 30 axial slices were taken with an inter-slice distance of 1 cm. On each of these slices, we use Canny Operator [3] for edge detection followed by GHT [1] for circle detection. The GHT is a model-based method for object localization utilizing a voting process to identify the likeliest position of the object of interest. Two circles with the strongest Hough-peaks were detected in each slice, and we consider they are mostly possible corresponded to the ascending and descending aorta.

GHT is a robust and powerful method for circle detection, but one drawback is that false object candidates are usually obtained too. In order to exclude false results, we use the k-means clustering algorithm [5] to spatially cluster the set of candidate points. k-means is an unsupervised clustering algorithm that can be efficiently and easily applied. We partition the candidates into three clusters here, the centers of the two largest clusters in terms of number of elements are considered as the approximate positions in the ascending and descending aorta, the third one is considered as the false candidates cluster.

2.3 Bayesian Tracking

The goal of a vessel tracking algorithm is to generate a chain of segments $x_0 \to x_1 \to x_2 \to \cdots$ that presents the vessel, where x_t denotes a set of model parameters. The Bayesian tracking method that we use here is similar to the work of Florin et al. [4] and Schaap et al. [10]. For the sake of completeness, we first briefly describe the basic Bayesian tracking. From a given starting point inside a tubular structure, multiple hypotheses of the current branch segment are investigated. According to the Bayesian rule, the posterior probability of the given hypothesis is estimated using a prior knowledge and likelihood information. A new hypothesis is created from a set of the most probable hypotheses. Upon successful propagation, the track with the maximal posterior probability is used to reconstruct the vessel. In our work, we want to use the unique aorta structure information that the centers of the ascending and descending aorta are getting closer when reaching the arch part. Therefore we incorporate the spatial distance changes between the ascending and descending aorta as another prior knowledge in the Bayesian method.

A tube is considered as a series of tube segments. A tube segment at iteration t is described by its location $p_t = (x_t, y_t, z_t)^T$, orientation $v_t = (\theta_t, \phi_t)$, radius r_t, intensity I_t, and the spatial distance between the ascending aorta and descending aorta d_t. Thus each tube segment is described by a state vector $x_t = (p_t, v_t, r_t, I_t, d_t)^T$. A vessel configuration is characterized by $x_{0:t} \equiv \{x_0, \cdots x_t\}$.

Based on the observation $z_{0:t}$ of the image data from iteration 0 to t, the posterior distribution measuring the fitness of the state vector $x_{0:t}$ with the corresponding observation $z_{0:t}$ can be estimated using the recursive Bayesian rule

$$p(x_{0:t}|z_{0:t}) \propto p(x_t|x_{t-1})p(z_t|x_t)p(x_{0:t-1}|z_{0:t-1}), \tag{1}$$

where $p(x_t|x_{t-1})$ denotes the prior probability and $p(z_t|x_t)$ denotes the likelihood function [10].

In the iteration step, the Bayesian rule incorporates the prior knowledge about the tubular structure into the tracking process. Using the manually identified centerlines from training datasets, distributions of radius changes, direction changes, and the spatial distance changes between the ascending and descending aorta are modeled as prior knowledge. We assume all the three variables are independent and Gaussian-distributed, and learn the respective means and standard deviations from 10 training datasets. More mathematical details can be found in [4] and [10].

2.4 Postprocessing

Sometimes the aortic arch is missing or partially occluded in a CT volume, and the two centerlines of ascending and descending aorta may not be spatially overlapped. So we estimate the approximate locations of the missing aortic arch segments in these scenarios in order to keep the completeness of the whole aorta centerline. We simply connect the two top points of the centerlines of the ascending and descending aorta.

3   Experiments and Results

3.1   Simulation Experiment

We first applied our automated method on simulated Dicom image datasets in various situations(see Fig. 4). Each dataset consists of 100 slices with pixel resolution of $1 \times 1 \times 1$ mm. The centerlines of the simulated aorta were tracked and the 3D models were reconstructed subsequently.

For evaluating our method, we compared the mean of the diameters on cross-section of the segmented aorta model to the known simulation values, and also calculate the differences of the corresponding centerline points between the automated tracked results and known model values (Table 1).

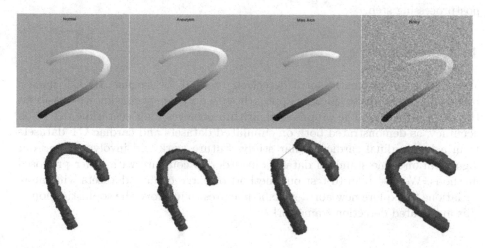

Fig. 4. Simulation experiments in various situations: normal image, aneurysm image, image with missing arch, image with Gaussian noise. The upper row are the simulation models; the lower row are the reconstructed results with centerline.

Table 1. Comparison of the automated results and model values.

Model	Normal	Aneurysm	Missing Arch	Noisy
Mean of cross-section diameter difference (mm)	0.08	0.07	0.09	1.08
Mean of centerline point difference (mm)	0.92	0.85	1.43	0.90

Table 2. The mean μ and standard deviation σ of the distance difference between the sample points on automated tracked and manually tracked centerlines.

	Ascending aorta	Aortic arch	Descending aorta	Whole aorta
Distance difference ($\mu \pm \sigma$) (mm)	1.8 ± 0.5	5.6 ± 1.9	1.5 ± 0.3	3.2 ± 1.2

3.2   Clinical Data Experiment

Experiments were conducted on cardiac CT exams of 34 subjects who are a part of a longitudinal cardiovascular study. Each exam contains about 200–300 CT slices with pixel resolution of 0.488 × 0.488 × 0.625 mm. Among these datasets, 10 exams were used to train the parameters for Bayesian tracking; 24 exams that do not belong to the training sets were used to test our automated algorithm.

To assess the accuracy of the method, we sampled a total of 60 points on the centerline in each case, and calculated the difference between these automated results and manually measured results. As shown in Table 2, there are high agreements between the automated and manual results. The aortic arch has the biggest difference because the arch is missing or partially missing in 9 exams, and their full centerlines were found based on some estimations in the postprocessing step.

4   Conclusion

We present an automatic aorta detection method for cardiac 3D CT images based on a probabilistic tracking approach with domain-specific knowledge about the aorta structure. The proposed algorithm achieves high centerline detection accuracy, as demonstrated both on simulated datasets and cardiac CT datasets from a longitudinal cardiovascular study. Future work will involve testing our algorithm on some standard datasets in order to compare with other proposed methods. We also plan to test our method on large clinical datasets with more variations to explore new aorta-specific features to improve the sophistication of this automated detection framework.

References

1. Ballard, D.H.: Generalizing the hough transform to detect arbitrary shapes. Pattern Recogn. **13**(2), 111–122 (1981)
2. Biesdorf, A., Worz, S., von Tengg-Kobligk, H., Rohr, K.: Automatic detection of supraaortic branches and model-based segmentation of the aortic arch from 3D CTA images. In: IEEE International Symposium on Biomedical Imaging: From Nano to Macro, 2009, ISBI'09, pp. 486–489. IEEE (2009)
3. Canny, J.: A computational approach to edge detection. IEEE Trans. Pattern Anal. Mach. Intell. **6**, 679–698 (1986)
4. Florin, C., Paragios, N., Williams, J.: Particle filters, a quasi-monte carlo solution for segmentation of coronaries. In: Duncan, J.S., Gerig, G. (eds.) MICCAI 2005. LNCS, vol. 3749, pp. 246–253. Springer, Heidelberg (2005)
5. Hartigan, J.A., Wong, M.A.: Algorithm as 136: a k-means clustering algorithm. J. Roy. Stat. Soc. Ser. C (Applied Statistics) **28**(1), 100–108 (1979)
6. Isgum, I., Staring, M., Rutten, A., Prokop, M., Viergever, M.A., van Ginneken, B.: Multi-atlas-based segmentation with local decision fusion application to cardiac and aortic segmentation in CT scans. IEEE Trans. Med. Imaging **28**(7), 1000–1010 (2009)

7. Lesage, D., Angelini, E.D., Bloch, I., Funka-Lea, G.: Medial-based bayesian tracking for vascular segmentation: application to coronary arteries in 3D CT angiography. In: 5th IEEE International Symposium on Biomedical Imaging: From Nano to Macro, 2008, ISBI 2008, pp. 268–271. IEEE (2008)

8. Manghat, N.E., Morgan-Hughes, G.J., Marshall, A.J., Roobottom, C.A.: Multi-detector row computed tomography: imaging the coronary arteries. Clin. Radiol. **60**(9), 939–952 (2005)

9. Phalla, O., Bonnet, D., Auriacombe, L., Pedroni, E., Balleux, F., Sidi, D., Mousseaux, E.: Late systemic hypertension and aortic arch geometry after successful repair of coarctation of the aorta. Eur. Heart J. **25**(20), 1853–1859 (2004)

10. Schaap, M., Smal, I., Metz, C.T., van Walsum, T.: Bayesian tracking of elongated structures in 3D images. In: Karssemeijer, N., Lelieveldt, B. (eds.) IPMI 2007. LNCS, vol. 4584, pp. 74–85. Springer, Heidelberg (2007)

11. Zhao, F., Zhang, H., Wahle, A., Scholz, T.D., Sonka, M.: Automated 4D segmentation of aortic magnetic resonance images. In: British Machine Vision Conference (BMVA), vol. 1, pp. 247–256 (2006)

12. Zheng, Y., John, M., Liao, R., Boese, J., Kirschstein, U., Georgescu, B., Zhou, S.K., Kempfert, J., Walther, T., Brockmann, G., Comaniciu, D.: Automatic aorta segmentation and valve landmark detection in C-arm CT: application to aortic valve implantation. In: Jiang, T., Navab, N., Pluim, J.P.W., Viergever, M.A. (eds.) MICCAI 2010, Part I. LNCS, vol. 6361, pp. 476–483. Springer, Heidelberg (2010)

Organ Localization Using Joint AP/LAT View Landmark Consensus Detection and Hierarchical Active Appearance Models

Qi Song[1], Albert Montillo[1]([✉]), Roshni Bhagalia[1], and V. Srikrishnan[2]

[1] General Electric Global Research, Niskayuna, NY, USA
[2] General Electric Global Research, Bangalore, India
{song,bhagalia,montillo}@ge.com

Abstract. Parsing 2D radiographs into anatomical regions is a challenging task with many applications. In the clinic, scans routinely include anterior-posterior (AP) and lateral (LAT) view radiographs. Since these orthogonal views provide complementary anatomic information, an integrated analysis can afford the greatest localization accuracy. To solve this integration we propose automatic landmark candidate detection, pruned by a learned geometric consensus detector model and refined by fitting a hierarchical active appearance organ model (H-AAM). Our main contribution is twofold. First, we propose a probabilistic joint consensus detection model which learns how landmarks in *either or both* views predict landmark locations in a given view. Second, we refine landmarks by fitting a joint H-AAM that learns how landmark arrangement and image appearance can help predict across views. This increases accuracy and robustness to anatomic variation. All steps require just seconds to compute and compared to processing the scouts separately, joint processing reduces mean landmark distance error from 27.3 mm to 15.7 mm in LAT view and from 12.7 mm to 11.2 mm in the AP view. The errors are comparable to human expert inter-observer variability and suitable for clinical applications such as personalized scan planning for dose reduction. We assess our method using a database of scout CT scans from 93 subjects with widely varying pathology.

Keywords: Automatic landmark localization · Organ localization · Image parsing · CT · Hierarchical active appearance model · Rejection cascade

1 Introduction

Many medical imaging protocols rely on 2-D radiographs for patient specific organ localization, which facilitates a variety of clinical applications including scanner set-up and scan planning, precise organ segmentation, semantic navigation and structured image search. Manual organ localization can be time consuming, impede workflow and often suffers from large operator errors. Automatic

---

Authors 'Q. Song' and 'A. Montillo' contributed equally.

B. Menze et al. (Eds.): MCV 2013, LNCS 8331, pp. 138–147, 2014.
DOI: 10.1007/978-3-319-05530-5_14, © Springer International Publishing Switzerland 2014

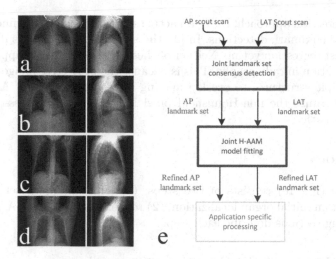

Fig. 1. Image analysis challenges and proposed solution. (a–d) Image paris consist of AP (left) and LAT (right) views. (e) Our method consists of two steps: joint landmark set detection followed by joint H-AAM organ localization.

localization from 2-D radiographs is therefore urgently needed. In this paper, we enable the automatic parsing of 2D radiographs from ubiquitous clinical CT scans. Such scans routinely include both a 2D anterior-posterior (AP) scout and a lateral (LAT) projection scout image. Automatic organ localization from 2-D scout images is a very challenging task due to low image quality from high noise level and low image contrast. Furthermore, scout images are 2-D projections of three dimensional data and as such have greatly reduced image information due to significant tissue overlap compared to volumetric scans. Representative 2D scout images are shown in Fig. 1a–d.

We hypothesize that an image analysis method combining information from AP and LAT views will afford the greatest localization accuracy. Our proposed solution (Fig. 1e) has two steps. First a set of landmarks delineating the boundaries of salient organs is extracted from the image pair though a joint consensus detector which removes outliers from the set of landmark candidates detected on AP *and* LAT views. This organ localization is further refined by fitting a hierarchical active appearance organ model (H-AAM) to the image pair.

Previous methods using landmark detection to parse radiographs include [5,8]. In [8] false negatives are not inferred nor are the detections refined with a joint H-AAM which we show substantially improve accuracy. In [5] the landmark detection uses only a single AP-only model and does not handle LAT images. It is essential to process both scouts because their orthogonal views provide complementary organ location information. Parsing 3D CT volumes using landmark detection has been presented [6], where the landmark detections are refined by searching exemplar cross-correlation maps. Active shape model (ASM) [3] and active appearance model (AAM) [1] have also been reported to combine with landmark detection approach. In [7], an active shape model based refinement was applied after landmark detections. In [2], the shape model fitting is driven by a random forest regression voting. Neither of these methods directly applies to soft tissue localization in radiographs. This is because the projective image formation causes multiple structures to overlap making direct application of ASMs error prone and because the non-Hounsfield pixel intensities make cross-correlation maps problematic.

2   Methods

Our method (Fig. 1e) consists of two steps: (1) joint landmark set consensus detection for an initial organ localization, (2) refinement by joint H-AAM fitting. The following sections describe each step.

2.1   Joint Landmark Set Detection

Joint landmark set detection consist of two substeps. We begin with the input which consists of a pair of 2D scout images, one for the AP scout, denoted I_{AP}, and one for the LAT scout, I_{LAT} (Fig. 2a). These are processed separately using an *individual "sliding-window" patch detector* for each landmark. One set of detectors searches I_{AP} and outputs a set of candidate landmark locations C_{AP}, while another set searches I_{LAT} and outputs candidate locations C_{LAT}. Detectors are run in parallel. In general, the output candidate sets contain false positives and negatives. Both are corrected by applying a *joint landmark set consensus detector* in Fig. 2a (box 3). This employs a greedy approach that iteratively removes the least likely candidate, considering the set of candidates recovered from both views and the probabilistic anatomy (landmark constellation) model. The result after consensus detection is a consistent N-labeling of the N landmarks for each subject. These N labels consist of landmarks for the AP scout, $L_{AP,1}$, and for the LAT scout $L_{LAT,1}$.

Training and Applying Landmark Detectors. Each individual landmark detector is trained as a two-category rejection cascade classifier [9], Fig. 2e, using supervised learning. Each cascade stage is a Gentle Adaboost [4] classifier.

To train we need positive landmark patches and negative patches. Positives come from cropping a rectangular patch around each manually annotated landmark. As illustrated in Fig. 2b we manually label 21 *AP landmarks* including: heart-diaphragm intersection (1, 11), diaphragm peak (2), lung corners (3, 19), left most in left lung (15), lung sides at 1/3 and 2/3 the arc length to top (4, 5, 18, 17), top of lungs (6, 16), airway-lung intersections (7, 13), heart top (14), heart sides (8, 12) at 1/2 arc length to top, ends of diaphragm near heart (9, 10), lower rib cage beneath lungs (20, 21). As shown in Fig. 2c we use 13 *LAT landmarks*: ends of diaphragm (1, 13), spine-diaphragm intersection (2), top of lung (5), lung side (3, 12) at 2/3 the arc length to top, posterior of spine (4) at 2/3 the arc length to lung top, heart top (6), heart side (7), heart-diaphragm intersection

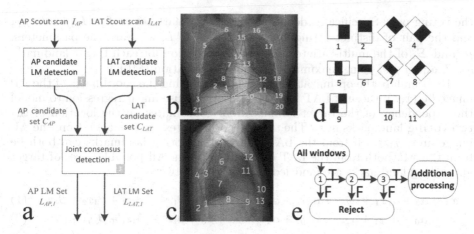

Fig. 2. Joint landmark set detection. (a) Landmark detectors scan input images producing landmark candidates; then a joint consensus detector corrects false positives and negatives. (b, c) Detectors are trained from positive and negative landmark patches dropped from images with manually labeled landmarks on lung and heart boundaries. (d) Haar image features (e) Rejection cascade based detectors.

(8), bottom of heart (9), right most of heart (10), heart side (11) at 2/3 the arc length bottom to top. These landmarks delineate lung and heart boundaries. The positive exemplars for each landmark are image patches large enough to include visible anatomical structure around the landmark. Negative exemplars are randomly cropped from the image that overlap the positive by $<40\%$. Haar image features (Fig. 2d) are computed efficiently using integral images [9]. Each cascade stage is trained to achieve a true positive rate of 99.7 % with a false positive rate of 50 % and stages are added until a desired overall true/false positive rate is reached or a maximum number of stages (15) is achieved.

Joint Landmark Set Consensus Detector. Applying the landmark detectors yields a set of candidate detections, $C = C_{AP} \cup C_{LAT}$. There can be multiple detections per landmark (false positives) and landmarks that were not detected but are present (false negatives). To correct for both cases we use a consensus detector to remove the false positives and infer the false negatives. There are two phases of consensus detection: training and application of the trained model which are described next.

Phase 1, Training: Training learns a probabilistic model of the global geometric arrangement of the landmarks in the N-landmark constellation. Given the manually labeled N-landmark set for each pair of training images, then for each **target** landmark i, and for each pair of **voting** landmarks from the remaining $N-1$, we learn the multivariate Gaussian distribution of the relative position of i to the location of the pair. Each distribution encodes the probability the target landmark i is at any location in the image plane, conditioned on the location of the voting pair. Specifically, denoting the N-landmark set as $L = L_{AP} \cup L_{LAT}$, and the pair of distinct voting landmarks as $s_i \subset L$, we learn the parameters, $\boldsymbol{\mu}_i$ and $\boldsymbol{\Sigma}_i$ of the multi-variate Gaussian distribution for each target landmark, $q \in L$ and $q \notin s_i$ using maximum likelihood estimation (MLE).

To formulate the optimization, we begin by letting the coordinates of the AP image be (x, z); those of LAT image be (y, z). We use linear regression to model the dependency of the target landmark q's coordinates on the location of the two **voting** landmarks in s_i. The target's coordinates are (x_3, z_3) if from the AP image and (y_3, z_3) if from the LAT image. The voting landmarks can both be from the AP, both from the LAT or one from each. All possible cases of target and voting landmarks are modeled using Eqs. (1)–(6):

$$x_3 = \alpha_0 + \alpha_1 x_1 + \alpha_2 z_1 + \alpha_3 x_2 + \alpha_4 z_2 \quad z_3 = \beta_0 + \beta_1 x_1 + \beta_2 z_1 + \beta_3 x_2 + \beta_4 z_2 \quad (1)$$

$$x_3 = \alpha_0 + \alpha_1 x_1 + \alpha_2 z_1 + \alpha_3 y_2 + \alpha_4 z_2 \quad z_3 = \beta_0 + \beta_1 x_1 + \beta_2 z_1 + \beta_3 y_2 + \beta_4 z_2 \quad (2)$$

$$x_3 = \alpha_0 + \alpha_1 y_1 + \alpha_2 z_1 + \alpha_3 y_2 + \alpha_4 z_2 \quad z_3 = \beta_0 + \beta_1 y_1 + \beta_2 z_1 + \beta_3 y_2 + \beta_4 z_2 \quad (3)$$

$$y_3 = \alpha_0 + \alpha_1 y_1 + \alpha_2 z_1 + \alpha_3 y_2 + \alpha_4 z_2 \quad z_3 = \beta_0 + \beta_1 y_1 + \beta_2 z_1 + \beta_3 y_2 + \beta_4 z_2 \quad (4)$$

$$y_3 = \alpha_0 + \alpha_1 y_1 + \alpha_2 z_1 + \alpha_3 x_2 + \alpha_4 z_2 \quad z_3 = \beta_0 + \beta_1 y_1 + \beta_2 z_1 + \beta_3 x_2 + \beta_4 z_2 \quad (5)$$

$$y_3 = \alpha_0 + \alpha_1 x_1 + \alpha_2 z_1 + \alpha_3 x_2 + \alpha_4 z_2 \quad z_3 = \beta_0 + \beta_1 x_1 + \beta_2 z_1 + \beta_3 x_2 + \beta_4 z_2 \quad (6)$$

Using the voting pair s_i, we model the probability that the target is at any location $\boldsymbol{x}$ in the kth training image as a multivariate Gaussian:

$$p_k(\boldsymbol{x}) = \frac{1}{\sqrt{2\pi |\boldsymbol{\Sigma}_{ki}|}} e^{-\frac{1}{2}(\boldsymbol{x} - \boldsymbol{\mu}_{ki})^T \boldsymbol{\Sigma}_{ki}^{-1}(\boldsymbol{x} - \boldsymbol{\mu}_{ki})}.$$

The unknown coefficients from the appropriate pair of linear regression equations (1)–(6) can be used to form a projection matrix:

$$\boldsymbol{A}_i = \begin{pmatrix} \alpha_0 & \beta_0 \\ \alpha_1 & \beta_1 \\ \alpha_2 & \beta_2 \\ \alpha_3 & \beta_3 \\ \alpha_4 & \beta_4 \end{pmatrix} \quad (7)$$

Similarly, given K total training LAT/AP image pairs, the coordinates of the voting landmarks can be expressed compactly as $\boldsymbol{P}_s$ (where x becomes x or y depending on AP or LAT) and the target coordinates as $\boldsymbol{P}_t$ using:

$$\boldsymbol{P}_s = \begin{pmatrix} 1 & x_{11} & z_{11} & x_{21} & z_{21} \\ 1 & x_{12} & z_{12} & x_{22} & z_{23} \\ \vdots & \vdots & \vdots & \vdots & \vdots \\ 1 & x_{1k} & z_{1k} & x_{2k} & z_{2k} \end{pmatrix} \quad (8)$$

$$\boldsymbol{P}_t = \begin{pmatrix} x_1 & x_2 & \dots & x_k \\ z_1 & z_2 & \dots & z_k \end{pmatrix} \quad (9)$$

We compute the projection matrix via MLE using $A_i = (P_s^T P_s)^{-1}(P_t P_s)^T$. Then the mean and covariance parameterizing the Gaussian are computed from: $\mu_i = P_s A_i$ and $\Sigma_i = cov(P_t^T - \mu_i)$. Note that even if the AP and LAT scans are not aligned well our method *still works well* because our model learns the distribution of AP/LAT misalignments.

Phase 2, application of the trained model: First we iteratively prune false positives, similar to [7,8]. At each iteration we remove the candidate least likely to be valid. Candidate likelihood is the maximum probability of the candidate, computed from the Gaussian distributions given its relative position to all other pairs of landmark candidates. Lowest probability candidate is removed if its probability is $<\tau$, an empirically determined threshold. Iterations stop when the lowest probability $>\tau$.

Next we infer the location of false negative landmarks, which is unique to our method and not found in [7,8]. Given C our set of candidate detections, we let P be the set of landmarks spanned by C. The undetected landmarks are $U = L \setminus P$. For each undetected landmark $u \in U$, we infer its location, x, using predictions from the detected candidates. We compute a location estimate for each subset $c_k \subset P$ of two candidates of distinct landmarks, using the mean offset, μ, from c_k learned in our training dataset. This forms a set of estimates, $E = \{e_n\}$ where $e_n = (x_n, z_n)$ for AP image. Our final estimate of e_n is formed from the trimmed mean of the central 50 % over all estimates in E.

2.2 Joint H-AAM Organ Localization

Joint H-AAM. Like the consensus detector, the active appearance model (AAM) is also a generative learning-based approach. Trained on labelled image data, the model learn both relative positions between different parts of the object and the expected textures inside the ROI. By incorporating both shape and appearance information, AAM-based interpretation leads to a robust solution even in the presence of serious image noise and large structure variation.

In this work, a joint H-AAM approach is introduced, encoding shape and appearance information from both AP and LAT views. Furthermore, a hierarchical pyramid is employed. At the coarse level, a single global joint model is trained on the manually-labelled radiographs of AP and LAT views. All landmarks used to train joint consensus detectors are included in the model. There are 21 landmarks in training image I_{AP} of AP scout and 13 landmarks in I_{LAT} of LAT scout. Through concatenation the shape of the training image pair is represented by a 34 dimensional vector $v = [L_{AP}, L_{LAT}]^T$, where $L_{AP} = [x_1^{AP}, z_1^{AP}, \cdots, x_{21}^{AP}, z_{21}^{AP}]$ is the set of 2D coordinates of landmarks in I_{AP} and $L_{LAT} = [y_1^{LAT}, z_1^{LAT}, ..., y_{13}^{LAT}, z_{13}^{LAT}]$ is the set for I_{LAT}. To obtain the associated appearance information, we construct two triangulated meshes based on these landmarks, one on AP view and one on LAT view (see Fig. 3a). The region inside the mesh is taken as the ROI. A global AAM model is then trained from the v and the ROI of the training images, which encodes the intensity texture from both AP and LAT scouts. Figure 3(b and c) show the constructed mean

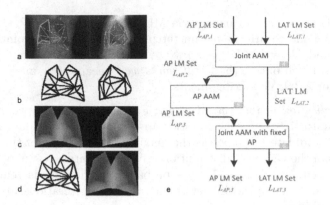

Fig. 3. (a) Triangulated meshes from manually-annotated landmarks give rough locations of lungs (green, blue, orange) and heart (red). (b) Mean joint shape model. (c) Mean joint appearance model. (d) Mean shape and appearance AP sub-model. (e) Joint H-AAM fitting workflow (Color figure online).

shape and the mean appearance of the joint model, respectively. The joint global model captures the probabilistic correlation between structures in both views, which helps infer obscured shapes from other parts and is less sensitive to initialization errors though less flexible than two individual scout models.

In subsequent finer levels of the pyramid, sub-models are trained using scout specific vertices from the global model, allowing better description of local structures and reducing the chance of over-constrained by learning variations in a single view. Figure 3d shows the constructed AP only sub-model. The following section shows how hierarchical model fitting helps localize organs in AP and LAT views.

Hierarchical Model Fitting. Our model fitting workflow is illustrated in Fig. 3e. Initialized to landmark consensus detection results, a joint model incorporating feature points from both AP and LAT scout images is simultaneously fitted to the AP/LAT image pair (Fig. 3e, box 4). Next the localization result on the AP image is refined by applying a sub-model learned from AP images, which is initialized by previous joint model fitting results (Fig. 3e, box 5). We only apply the sub-model for AP scouts because in practice, AP images have more reliable features since the projection image is formed from less tissue overlap than LAT images. Since LAT images have greater structure occlusion more constraints are required to infer organ locations. To further refine LAT locations, we fit a joint model again, during which we leave the AP landmarks fixed. These points serve as reliable "anchor" points, enforcing contextual constraints for LAT landmark refinement.

3   Experiments and Results

We evaluate our approach on 93 subjects from whom both AP and LAT scout images were acquired using four-fold cross validation, i.e. 70 subjects for training and the remainder for testing in each fold. The image size ranges from 888×660 pixels to 888×1026 pixels for AP scout, and 888×660 pixels to 888×935 pixels for LAT scout. The resolution is 0.60×0.55 mm for both scouts. The subjects vary in age, gender, and pathology including obesity (Fig. 1b), lung cancer, and cardiomyopathy. Additional variability includes metallic implants: cardiac stents, hip implants, and jewelry (Fig. 1a, c). Acquisition protocol variations include large variation in the Z range and patient positioning, e.g. arm position (Fig. 1a, d).

Qualitative Evaluation. In Fig. 4a, we compare landmark detection results using separate consensus detection, (top), with those from joint consensus detection, (bottom). True landmarks are shown in dark blue X's, those detected by the method are shown as green and yellow X's, while those inferred using these detections are light blue. Differences are highlighted in yellow; the detection and the corresponding true location are enclosed by a yellow ellipse. We observe these ellipses are much smaller using joint consensus detection than separate detection, indicating higher landmark accuracy. In further analysis we found that every LAT landmark has improved mean accuracy. Figure 4b–d show comparative organ localization results. The fitting results are shown in cyan dashes with right lung (green), left lung (blue), chest cavity (orange) and heart (red). The ground-truth is marked by yellow dash. We observe the joint model yields significant improvement (Fig. 4c) over the single view processing (Fig. 4b) and is further improved by enforcing a joint hierarchical model fitting structure (Fig. 4d).

Quantitative Evaluation. The mean landmark distance error between computed and manually labelled landmarks across all 93 test images is shown in Fig. 5a. Compared to separate view consensus detection, our proposed joint view approach reduces distance error from 12.7 mm to 11.2 mm for AP view and from 27.3 mm to 15.7 mm for LAT view. Joint consensus detection without AAM fitting maintains AP landmarks at 22.3 mm while dramatically reducing error (by >14 mm) for LAT view from 32.0 mm to 17.3 mm. Joint *hierarchical* AAM reduces overall distance error for *AP and LAT*, including from 14.0 mm to 11.2 mm for AP and from 17.3 mm to 15.7 mm for LAT compared to joint model fitting only.

A potential application of our method is to determine the bounding box of the heart for cardiac scan range planning. To evaluate method suitability we compare the smallest rectangle containing all landmarks along the heart boundary to heart bounding boxes manually defined by physicians. The unsigned distance errors of the box sides are shown in Fig. 5b–c. Our method improves bottom and all four sides in AP and LAT scouts respectively. Improvement of the bottom side is particularly noteworthy given the high organ occlusion there.

Processing the images at full resolution, landmark detection and joint consensus detection takes about 25 s while joint H-AAM requires about 30 s with a modern desktop computer (4–8 core, 8 GB RAM). Further speedup is achievable through multi-resolution processing.

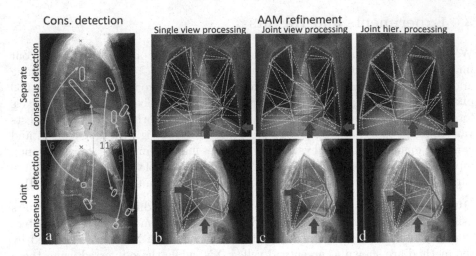

Fig. 4. Impact of joint AP/LAT view processing. (a) Separate detection results (top) have larger landmark errors than joint consensus detection (bottom) for landmarks (red #). (b)–(d) Each step in which we fit our AAM model (shown with red, blue, green, cyan lines) improves fidelity to ground-truth (yellow dash). Compare fitting improvements (purple arrows) among (b) single view AAM; (c) joint view AAM and (d) joint H-AAM (Color figure online).

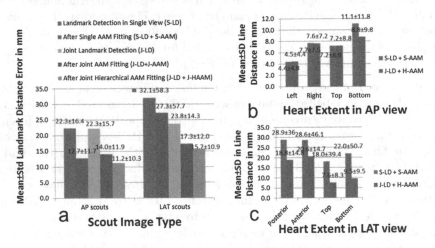

Fig. 5. Cross-validation results from 93 subjects. Proposed joint AP/LAT view approach achieves lowest distance error (a) and heart bounding-box distance error (b, c).

4   Discussion and Conclusions

In this work we address the challenging task of parsing AP and LAT radiographs into salient anatomic structures. To the best of our knowledge, *this work is the first to jointly leverage information from AP and LAT scouts to delineate the heart and lungs.* We demonstrate that fitting a coarser initial joint hierarchical AAM across AP/LAT views reliably refines the consensus landmark detection results. Further, finer single-view-only models can be subsequently applied for a final round of refinement. Using joint landmark detection and joint H-AAM fitting reduces mean distance error in LAT landmarks from 27.3 to 15.7 mm. This is an improvement of over 40 percent compared to using only LAT scout scans, where features are inherently more difficult to localize due to greater overlap of structures. Lastly, compared to separate view processing, our joint view approach reduces overall mean landmark distance error from 12.7 mm to 11.2 mm in the AP view and from 27.3 mm to 15.7 mm in LAT view. For the AP scout our error of 11.2 mm compares well to the mean human expert inter-observer variability of 10.2 mm while our error for the LAT scout of 15.7 mm compares to the human inter-observer error of 14.3 mm. These inter observer errors were computed using manual landmark estimates obtained from two independent observers. Our algorithm achieves a level of accuracy sufficient to enable clinically relevant tasks such as reducing radiation for the patient through personalized scan planning and to facilitate consistent longitudinal scanning in the clinic, and such clinical productization has already begun.

References

1. Cootes, T., Edwards, G., Taylor, C.: Active appearance models. IEEE Trans. Pattern Anal. Mach. Intell. **23**(6), 681–685 (2001)
2. Cootes, T.F., Ionita, M.C., Lindner, C., Sauer, P.: Robust and accurate shape model fitting using random forest regression voting. In: Fitzgibbon, A., Lazebnik, S., Perona, P., Sato, Y., Schmid, C. (eds.) ECCV 2012, Part VII. LNCS, vol. 7578, pp. 278–291. Springer, Heidelberg (2012)
3. Cootes, T., Taylor, C., Cooper, D., Graham, J.: Active shape models-their training and application. Comput. Vis. Image Underst. **61**(1), 38–59 (1995)
4. Freund, Y., Schapire, R.: Experiments with a new boosting algorithm. In: Saitta, L. (ed.) ICML, pp. 148–156. Morgan Kaufmann, San Francisco (1996)
5. Montillo, A., Song, Q., Liu, X., Miller, J.: Parsing radiographs by integrating landmark set detection and multi-object active appearance models. SPIE Medical Imaging (2013)
6. Potesil, V., Kadir, T., Platsch, G., Brady, M.: Personalization of pictorial structures for anatomical landmark localization. In: Székely, G., Hahn, H.K. (eds.) IPMI 2011. LNCS, vol. 6801, pp. 333–345. Springer, Heidelberg (2011)
7. Seifert, S., Barbu, A., Zhou, S., Liu, D., Feulner, J., Huber, M., Suehling, M., Cavallaro, A., Comaniciu, D.: Hierarchical parsing and semantic navigation of full body CT data. SPIE Med. Imaging **7259**, 02:1–8 (2009)
8. Tao, Y., Peng, Z., Krishnan, A., Zhou, X.: Robust learning-based parsing and annotation of medical radiographs. IEEE Trans. Med. Imaging **30**(2), 338–350 (2011)
9. Viola, P., Jones, M.: Robust real-time face detection. IJCV **57**(2), 137–154 (2004)

Pectoral Muscle Detection in Digital Breast Tomosynthesis and Mammography

Florin C. Ghesu[1,2]($\boxtimes$), Michael Wels[1], Anna Jerebko[3], Michael Sühling[1], Joachim Hornegger[2], and B. Michael Kelm[1]

[1] Siemens Corporate Technology, Imaging and Computer Vision,
Erlangen, Germany
florin.c.ghesu@fau.de
[2] Pattern Recognition Chair, Friedrich Alexander University,
Erlangen, Germany
[3] Siemens AG, Healthcare, Erlangen, Germany

Abstract. Screening and diagnosis of breast cancer with Digital Breast Tomosynthesis (DBT) and Mammography are increasingly supported by algorithms for automatic post-processing. The pectoral muscle, which dorsally delineates the breast tissue towards the chest wall, is an important anatomical structure for navigation. Along with the nipple and the skin, the pectoral muscle boundary is often used for reporting the location of breast lesions. It is visible in mediolateral oblique (MLO) views where it is well approximated by a straight line. Here, we propose two machine learning-based algorithms to robustly detect the pectoral muscle in MLO views from DBT and mammography. Embedded into the Marginal Space Learning framework, the algorithms involve the evaluation of multiple candidate boundaries in a hierarchical manner. To this end, we propose a novel method for candidate generation using a Hough-based approach. Experiments were performed on a set of 100 DBT volumes and 95 mammograms from different clinical cases. Our novel combined approach achieves competitive accuracy and robustness. In particular, for the DBT data, we achieve significantly lower deviation angle error and mean distance error than the standard approach. The proposed algorithms run within a few seconds.

1 Introduction

Breast cancer has the highest incidence rate among cancerous diseases affecting women (2008 World Cancer Report[1]). Early diagnosis improves the effectiveness of treatment and is supported by comprehensive screening techniques, which are widely used from earliest disease stages. In this context, 2D mammography with mediolateral oblique (MLO) and craniocaudal (CC) views is most widely employed. Recent advances in the diagnostic field introduce Digital Breast Tomosynthesis (DBT) as a diagnostic tool and potential screening alternative. The modality performs a high resolution 3D reconstruction from multiple

---

[1] http://globocan.iarc.fr

B. Menze et al. (Eds.): MCV 2013, LNCS 8331, pp. 148–157, 2014.
DOI: 10.1007/978-3-319-05530-5_15, © Springer International Publishing Switzerland 2014

2D angular projections. While both views, MLO and CC, can be acquired with DBT as well, very often, one MLO acquisition is sufficient due to the inherent 3D information.

Semi-automatic and automatic approaches for analyzing mammography and DBT frequently require the pectoral muscle boundary, which is a comparatively stable anatomical entity in MLO breast images. In computer-aided detection, for example, the breast tissue, which is dorsally bounded by the pectoral muscle, needs to be segmented [4]. As a second example, reporting can be automated by computing distances of detected lesions to the pectoral muscle (as well as the nipple). Finally, the pectoral muscle boundary can also be used for the registration of different views and modalities to support linked navigation [10,11].

Figure 1 shows examples of both imaging modalities. The sought boundary is mainly visible through faint lines and texture differences in the upper left part of the images. In addition to appearance characteristics, prior knowledge, assuming a correct image acquisition according to the existing quality standards, can be taken into account. In an optimal MLO view the pectoral muscle is usually located craniodorsal, extending to or below the posterior nipple line (the horizontal line through the nipple). In our work we employ a straight line model, with the main focus on the robustness of the detection process. This approximation is sufficient in many applications. If required, more refined approximations, such as the curvilinear delineation proposed in [1], may also gain from a robust straight line initialization. A reliable automatic detection of the pectoral muscle, however, faces several challenges such as inherent blurring or superimposed boundaries that are likely to compromise the final result (Fig. 1).

To overcome these challenges, we propose to apply Marginal Space Learning (MSL) [12], a machine learning-based methodology for robust detection. The MSL approach is extended by an algorithm based on the Hough transform [4]. Experiments were performed on an extensive data set and cross validation was

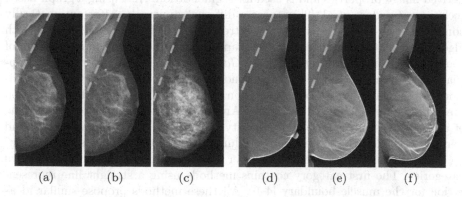

(a)   (b)   (c)   (d)   (e)   (f)

Fig. 1. Exemplary images with annotations. (a) and (b): mammograms containing superimposed boundaries (i.e. skin folds); (c): mammogram showing high intensity blurring; (d): transversal tomosynthesis slice with high smoothness in the structure; (e) and (f): DBT slices with intensity variation.

used to assess the detection accuracy and compare against the standard app-roach described in reference [4]. While the standard approach works well for mammography, its performance severely degrades on DBT data, which is proba-bly due to different contrasts that would require modifications of some heuristic parts of the algorithm. Different from that, our learning-based algorithms exhibit excellent and stable performance on both, DBT and mammography.

After a short review of related work in Sect. 2, we describe the Hough transform-based standard approach, the proposed marginal space learning app-roach and a novel combination of both in Sect. 3. An experimental evaluation and discussion is presented in Sect. 4, followed by a conclusion in Sect. 5.

2   Related Work

The problem of finding a precise pectoral muscle boundary in MLO mam-mograms has undergone considerable research, recently, for example, in refer-ences [1–3,5–7] and [8]. However, to the best of our knowledge there are no methods solving this problem specifically for DBT. For location mapping in ipsilateral breast tomosynthesis views, van Schie et al. [10] attempt pectoral muscle detection by using the standard *Hough transform*, an approach intro-duced by Karssemeijer [4] that was only evaluated on 2D mammograms. Using this background, Kinoshita et al. [5] propose a similar methodology applying the *Canny filter* and *Radon transform* to generate boundary candidates. Then a sim-ple heuristic is applied to support the decision for the target solution. Different from that, Bajger et al. [1] use the concept of *Minimum spanning tree* to model the distinct image segments. This information is then used to compute a curve which represents the target shape. An extension of this method is presented in the work of Ma and Bajger et al. [7] which is compared to another graph based approach using a multiresolution description of the image encoded in a multilayer graph. The connectivity between layers is based on image intensities as well as derived image properties and is used for segmentation. Also using a graph based technique, Cardoso et al. [2] propose a different approach. After automatically computing two control points on the extremity of the boundary, a shortest path algorithm is employed on a weighted graph derived from the polar transform of the mammogram. Ferrari et al. [3] use *Gabor wavelets* in a multiresolution app-roach considering the phase and magnitude images by employing vector summa-tion. Subsequent to a phase propagation, pixels with opposite phase direction are identified as boundary descriptors. Another method is presented by Sultana et al. [8] who estimate probability density functions of certain image points and perform classification and merge procedures to achieve a reliable segmentation.

All these approaches, along with other variants found in literature, define two categories. The first category contains methods using a straight line represen-tation for the muscle boundary [4–6]. All these methods propose similar ideas or variations from the algorithm described by Karssemeijer [4], which we use as reference in this work. The other category includes approaches employing a curvilinear detection. Due to differences in representation, a comparison between our approach and these methods is not possible.

3   Methods

For a self-contained presentation we first review pectoral muscle detection based on the Hough transform as proposed by Karssemeijer [4]. Then we describe line detection using MSL [12] and finally, a Hough-based candidate generation method within the MSL framework is proposed.

3.1   Hough Transform Approach

The reference approach [4] considered in this paper employs a constrained *Hough transform* to locate the pectoral muscle boundary. The detection procedure is based on the gradient image and divides into three major steps. First, the accumulator field over angle θ and radius ρ is computed. For this purpose the polar coordinates representation $\rho = x \cos \theta + y \sin \theta$ is used, where x and y are the Cartesian coordinates of the considered pixel and the angle parameter θ is evaluated within $\pm 9°$ of the local image gradient. In the second step, the accumulator field is modified to avoid a bias towards longer boundary lines and to eliminate solutions not lying within the expected region of interest (see Fig. 2). Finally, a peak detection heuristic is applied to either identify a viable pectoral muscle boundary or exclude its existence.

While the method performs well on full-field digital mammograms, its application to DBT exhibits weaknesses. Despite careful tuning of the heuristic threshold parameters, a comparable performance cannot be achieved on DBT as shown in Sect. 4. This is probably due to the fact that the pectoral muscle boundary is less pronounced in DBT and looks different from mammography (see Fig. 1).

3.2   Marginal Space Learning Approach

To resolve these issues, we propose to apply MSL [12], a robust supervised learning approach which tackles detection by solving an equivalent hierarchy of classification problems. The challenge of identifying the muscle boundary is

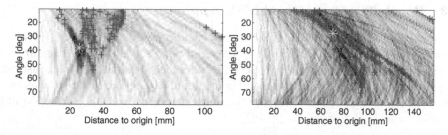

Fig. 2. Left: inverted accumulator field for mammogram showing one main cluster of labeled peaks (local maxima, *red* +); Right: inverted accumulator field for DBT slice showing a sparse distribution of the local maxima. The labeled local optima are in both plots larger than a certain threshold. The target solution is denoted by ∗ *(yellow)* (Color figure online).

thus reduced to decisions of classifiers on candidate solutions. While the original MSL approach is applied to object localization which includes position, orientation and scale of the sought object, here, we are interested in detecting straight lines.

The line detection problem is tackled with MSL by representing lines as position-orientation tuples (P_x, P_y, ϕ) ('boxes'), where ϕ denotes the angle and (P_x, P_y) a position on the line. While every such tuple uniquely represents a line, any line can be represented by an arbitrary number of such tuples due to the ambiguity of the position (P_x, P_y). This apparent drawback of the line representation is exploited by MSL which, by design, can perfectly handle solutions represented by multiple candidate tuples [12]. In fact, lines detected by the proposed MSL approach need to be supported by the majority of the most likely candidate tuples which assure optimal support in the analyzed image data (see Fig. 5c). For training, ground truth tuples are generated from the annotated straight line boundaries by equidistant sampling. In the same way, such tuples are generated from candidate lines provided by the Hough-based method as described in Sect. 3.3 (see Fig. 5b).

Figure 3 provides a schematic overview of the employed MSL pipeline which uses two detection stages. First, a number of likely candidate positions (P_x, P_y) are identified using a first classifier. These are then augmented with a discrete number of hypothesis angles to generate position-orientation candidate tuples (P_x, P_y, ϕ) which, are evaluated by a second classifier. Finally, the N ($N = 50$) most likely candidate tuples are aggregated to generate a unique solution. While this final step could encompass clustering and outlier removal (e.g. in Hough space), or methods from robust statistics, we only employed simple averaging in this work. In our experiments, we used Probabilistic Boosting-Trees (PBT) [9] along with Haar-like and steerable features [12] to capture position and orientation information in the underlying image data.

In addition to this approach, we also propose a way to incorporate the representation of lines in Hough space into the MSL framework as an alternative method for candidate generation.

3.3   Hough Transform-Based MSL Approach

A slight modification of the Hough-based method presented in Sect. 3.1 allows to generate multiple candidate lines instead of only one solution. In particular, the original peak selection heuristic proposed in reference [4] is omitted and, instead, the N biggest local optima in the modified accumulator field are extracted as candidate lines (see Fig. 5a). Candidate tuples are generated from the corresponding

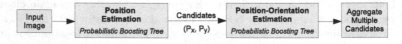

Fig. 3. Marginal Space Learning detection pipeline showing a cascade of two detectors.

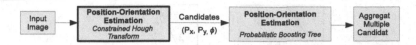

Fig. 4. Detection pipeline for combined approach. The standard PBT based position estimation is replaced by a modified Hough transform based detector.

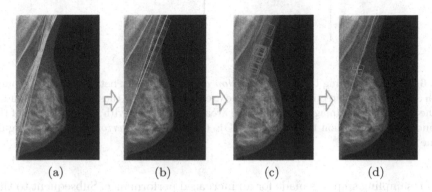

Fig. 5. Detection pipeline of the combined approach. (a): candidate lines corresponding to the top 25 peaks in Hough space. (b): isotropic boxes of size 16×16 mm are equidistantly generated along all candidate lines (visualization includes only 3 lines for clarity) and are subject to classification. (c): top 20 candidates of the PBT based position-orientation estimation. (d): ground truth *(orange dashed line)* and aggregated box detection along with the corresponding detection line *(green)* (Color figure online).

candidate lines by equidistant sampling within the image domain as exemplified in Fig. 5b. These candidate tuples are then evaluated by a joint position-orientation detector (see Fig. 5c). Finally, the top N candidates ($N = 50$) are averaged to generate the final solution (see Fig. 5d). Hence, compared to the MSL approach described in Sect. 3.2 (see Fig. 3), the original position detector is replaced by the Hough-based candidate generation method as shown in Fig. 4.

Note that, for this method to work, it is important to extract a sufficiently high number of candidates from the accumulator field to ensure that the correct solution is included (see Fig. 5a). The optimal number of candidates can be determined empirically, ranging in our experiments between 100–150 candidates for mammography and 350–400 candidates for DBT.

4   Experiments

To accurately assess the performance of the proposed algorithms we used representative data sets from different clinical cases for each image modality. 95 digital mammograms with an initial size of 2106×2740 pixels were resampled from a isotropic resolution of 0.085 mm to a target resolution of 1.5 mm. Furthermore, we extracted central transversal slices from 100 DBT volumes with a size of 1652×2820 pixels which were resampled to 1 mm isotropic resolution.

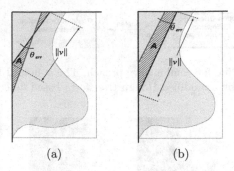

Fig. 6. Images depicting the DAE (*deviation angle error*) θ_{err} between the red ground truth and the green detection, as well as the area A spanned by these two lines (bounded by the left and upper image margins). The area is normalized with the length $\|v\|$ of the ground truth annotation to define the MDE (*mean distance error*) d_{err} (Color figure online).

This resampling step was made for an increased performance. Subsequent to this pre-processing stage, each image has been annotated by an experienced radiologist with the straight ground truth boundary line of the pectoral muscle. For all our experiments we used *10-fold cross validation* to assess the quality of the algorithms on unseen data. Statistical significance has been evaluated using a *paired T-test*.

For the assessment of the detection accuracy we employed two error measures. The first error measure is the *deviation angle error* (DAE) θ_{err}, which is the angular difference between the detected line u and the annotated reference v (see Fig. 6a). Since the DAE can be small despite a huge parallel displacement between detection and annotation (see Fig. 6b), we also define the *mean distance error* (MDE) d_{err}. This is computed as the area A spanned by the lines u and v, bounded by the left and upper image margins and normalized with the length $\|v\|$ of the annotated reference (see Fig. 6). Note that while DAE is invariant to scale and translation, MDE is designed to be sensitive to such operations, yielding a direct dependency to the position (implicitly length) of the lines. Thus, the two error measures are

$$\theta_{err} = \arccos\left(\frac{u \cdot v}{\|u\|\|v\|}\right) \quad \text{and} \quad d_{err} = \frac{A}{\|v\|} \ . \tag{1}$$

These two measures are combined to express the accuracy of a detection, generalized for the entire data set in a series of statistical markers. These are shown in Table 1 for both measures and all considered approaches. While specific values may indicate increased robustness of the combined approach on mammography (see DAE standard deviation: 2.891° and 95 % quantile: 8.32°), the employed statistical test (paired t-Test) reveals that the quality differences are not significant on this type of data (*p-value* > 0.05). However, the high stability of our proposed framework comes as a fundamental advantage against the standard approach. Being a learning based method, it can automatically adapt to

Table 1. Table showing in the upper part the *deviation angle error* (DAE) statistics for mammograms and DBT. All values are measured in degrees. The lower table lists the *mean distance error* (MDE), expressed in millimeters. While quality differences between the 3 approaches are not significant on mammography data, on DBT, both proposed learning based methods yield a significant improvement (*p-value* < 0.01) of the results from reference [4] (column *Hough*).

		Mammography			Digital Breast Tomosynthesis		
		Hough	MSL	Combination	Hough	MSL	Combination
DAE	Mean	3.106	3.612	2.426	7.857	2.692	3.149
	Standard deviation	3.708	6.187	2.891	13.636	2.495	4.573
	Median	1.675	2.521	1.547	2.999	1.890	1.649
	95 % quantile	12.716	8.479	8.320	45.508	8.078	12.868
MDE	Mean	6.517	6.433	3.934	9.799	2.612	3.049
	Standard deviation	12.649	14.835	7.953	16.685	3.348	4.270
	Median	2.760	2.638	2.018	2.049	1.681	1.503

any contrast variations that may result from different pre-processing strategies or acquisition setups. The generality of our approach applies also on DBT data. Here, the aforementioned challenges as well as additional diversity in the applied reconstruction techniques come as a serious impediment against the accuracy of threshold based methods (e.g. reference [4]).

Thus, on DBT, the two proposed novel approaches show a statistically significant performance gain (*p-value* < 0.01) achieving both a very low mean and standard deviation for both measures. The significant accuracy increase is also confirmed by the 95 % quantile of 8°, which is an indicator for the high robustness. While a close comparison of the two methods may show improvement tendencies of the MSL approach on DBT (w.r.t. MDE mean: 2.612 compared to 3.049 supposedly attributed to the impaired performance of the Hough Transform on this type of data), these differences are not statistically significant. This is a confirmation of the high performance stability of the two proposed algorithms (especially on DBT but also on mammography using the combined approach). Figure 7 shows detection results on various images from both modalities. The presented images show some of the challenges confronted by detection process (e.g. texture variation, blurring or superimposed boundaries).

A careful analysis of the proposed approaches shows that the accuracy of the final result is affected by the number of candidates used for aggregation. Figure 8 shows how the detection accuracy changes with the number of candidates, revealing the fact that optimal results are achieved with a number of candidates in the local neighborhood of 50 (on both mammography and DBT). Variations from this empirically chosen minimum point towards other local minima (see Fig. 8) may improve the accuracy by less than 0.2° (DAE) or 0.3 mm (MDE), differences which are considered to be negligible. The plots also show the general tendency of the mean and median to increase beyond 70 candidates, an observation which supports our choice for the optimum point. Both proposed

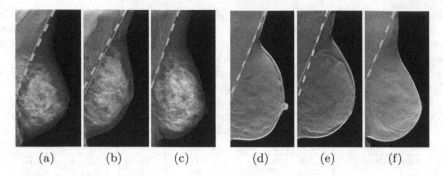

(a)   (b)   (c)   (d)   (e)   (f)

Fig. 7. Example images showing detection result *(green line)* and ground truth annotation *(orange dashed line)*. (a)–(c): mammograms yielding robust detections of the
combined method. (d)–(f): central, transversal DBT slices showing detection results of
the MSL approach. The accuracy of the detection is particularly high despite the high
smoothness in figure (d) or high intensity variations in figure (f) (Color figure online).

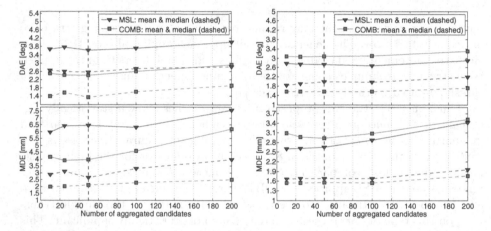

Fig. 8. Performance graphs showing compared accuracy variation with increasing number of aggregated candidates on mammography (left subfigure) and DBT (right subfigure). The plots show the variation for mean and median DAE as well as MDE for
both MSL (marginal space learning approach) and COMB (combined method).

methods run within about 3 s on a 2.2 GHz dual core machine which is in the
same range as the reference method from [4].

5   Conclusion

We presented a novel approach for the detection of the pectoral muscle boundary
that combines the previously applied Hough transform-based method and the
MSL framework. Detailed experiments have shown that result improvements are
significant on DBT data. Moreover, the framework can be successfully applied on

DBT slices and mammograms alike. To the best of our knowledge, this is the first reported system focused on supporting an effective, automatic pectoral muscle detection in DBT. Since the approach is learning-based it can easily be adapted to different contrasts which may result from diverse vendor-specific reconstruction and post-processing strategies. Also, the proposed approaches are fast and run within only a few seconds. Thus, they can readily be applied to enable automated measurements, navigation support through multimodal registration and computer-aided detection in the breast.

References

1. Bajger, M., Ma, F., Bottema, M.J.: Minimum spanning trees and active contours for identification of the pectoral muscle in screening mammograms. In: Proceedings of the Digital Image Computing on Techniques and Applications, pp. 47–51 (2005)
2. Cardoso, J.S., Domingues, I., Amaral, I., Moreira, I., Passarinho, P., Santa Comba, J., Correia, R., Cardoso, M.J.: Pectoral muscle detection in mammograms based on polar coordinates and the shortest path. IEEE Eng. Med. Biol. Soc. **2010**, 4781–4784 (2010)
3. Ferrari, R.J., Rangayyan, R.M., Desautels, J.E.L., Borges, R.A., Frere, A.F.: Automatic identification of the pectoral muscle in mammograms. IEEE Trans. Med. Imaging **23**, 232–245 (2004)
4. Karssemeijer, N.: Automated classification of parenchymal patterns in mammograms. Phys. Med. Biol. **43**, 365–378 (1998)
5. Kinoshita, S.K., Azevedo-Marques, P.M., Pereira Jr, R., Rodrigues, J.A.H., Rangayyan, R.M.: Radon-domain detection of the nipple and the pectoral muscle in mammograms. J. Digit. Imaging **21**, 37–49 (2008)
6. Kwok, S.M., Chandrasekhar, R., Attikiouzel, Y., Rickard, M.T.: Automatic pectoral muscle segmentation on mediolateral oblique view mammograms. IEEE Trans. Med. Imaging **23**, 1129–1140 (2004)
7. Ma, F., Bajger, M., Slavotinek, J.P., Bottema, M.J.: Two graph theory based methods for identifying the pectoral muscle in mammograms. Pattern Recogn. **40**, 2592–2602 (2007)
8. Sultana, A., Ciuc, M., Strungaru, R.: Detection of pectoral muscle in mammograms using a mean-shift segmentation approach. In: 8th International Conference on Communications, pp. 165–168 (2010)
9. Tu, Z.: Probabilistic boosting-tree: learning discriminative models for classification, recognition, and clustering. In: Proceedings of the Tenth IEEE International Conference on Computer Vision, vol. 2, pp. 1589–1596 (2005)
10. van Schie, G., Tanner, C., Snoeren, P., Samulski, M., Leifland, K., Wallis, M.G., Karssemeijer, N.: Correlating locations in ipsilateral breast tomosynthesis views using an analytical hemispherical compression model. Phys. Med. Biol. **56**, 4715–4730 (2011)
11. Wels, M., Kelm, B.M., Hammon, M., Jerebko, A., Sühling, M., Comaniciu, D.: Data-driven breast decompression and lesion mapping from digital breast tomosynthesis. In: Ayache, N., Delingette, H., Golland, P., Mori, K. (eds.) MICCAI 2012, Part I. LNCS, vol. 7510, pp. 438–446. Springer, Heidelberg (2012)
12. Zheng, Y., Georgescu, B., Comaniciu, D.: Marginal space learning for efficient detection of 2D/3D anatomical structures in medical images. In: Prince, J.L., Pham, D.L., Myers, K.J. (eds.) IPMI 2009. LNCS, vol. 5636, pp. 411–422. Springer, Heidelberg (2009)

Features and Retrieval

Computer Aided Diagnosis Using Multilevel Image Features on Large-Scale Evaluation

Le Lu[1,3]($\boxtimes$), Pandu Devarakota[2], Siddharth Vikal[2], Dijia Wu[3,4],
Yefeng Zheng[3], and Matthias Wolf[2]

[1] National Institutes of Health, Bethesda, USA
[2] Siemens Medical Solutions USA, Malvern, USA
[3] Siemens Corporate Research, Princeton, USA
[4] Microsoft Corporation, Redmond, USA
le.lu@nih.gov, mwolf@siemens.com

Abstract. Computer aided diagnosis (CAD) of cancerous anatomical structures via 3D medical images has emerged as an intensively studied research area. In this paper, we present a principled three-tiered image feature learning approach to capture task specific and data-driven class discriminative statistics from an annotated image database. It integrates voxel-, instance-, and database-level feature learning, aggregation and parsing. The initial segmentation is proceeded as robust voxel labeling and thresholding. After instance-level spatial aggregation, extracted features can also be flexibly tuned for classifying lesions, or discriminating different subcategories of lesions. We demonstrate the effectiveness in the lung nodule detection task which **handles all types of solid, partial-solid, and ground-glass nodules using the same set of learned features**. Our hierarchical feature learning framework, which was extensively trained and validated on large-scale multiple site datasets of 879 CT volumes (510 training and 369 validation), achieves superior performance than other state-of-the-art CAD systems. The proposed method is also shown to be applicable for **colonic polyp detection, including all polyp morphological subcategories**, via 770 tagged-prep CT scans from multiple medical sites (358 training and 412 validation).

1 Introduction

Lung cancer is the leading deadly cancer in western population, but similar to colon cancer, it is highly preventable if lung nodules can be detected early. Therefore, image-interpretation-based cancer detection using 3D computer tomography (CT) has emerged as a common clinical practice, and computer-aided detection tools for enhancing radiologists' diagnostic performance and effectiveness have been developed in the last decade. The key for radiologists to accept the clinical usage of a CAD system is the highest possible true positive (TP) detection sensitivity with the desirably low false positive (FP) rate per patient. In this paper, we exploit a new method of multilevel (discriminatively trained) image feature learning, as the key to achieve this goal.

B. Menze et al. (Eds.): MCV 2013, LNCS 8331, pp. 161–174, 2014.
DOI: 10.1007/978-3-319-05530-5_16, © Springer International Publishing Switzerland 2014

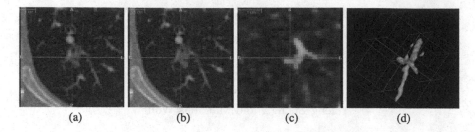

(a)   (b)   (c)   (d)

Fig. 1. Examples of training data and voxelwise annotation (Red for nodule; Green for vessel). (a) CT image displaying a Ground-Glass nodule; (b) its corresponding annotation; (c) CT image of a branching vessel with its annotation overlaid; (d) 3D volume rendering of the same structure to demonstrate its spatial complexity (Color figure online).

Many CAD algorithms highly depend on delicate lesion image segmentation algorithms to delineate the boundary of lesion tissue from its normal context surroundings in 2D/3D images. A collection of drastically different methods [1–3] have been proposed. The technical analogies of all methods are based on *analyzing low-level, surface geometric and volumetric intensity patterns*, and *exploiting strong spatial regularization* (e.g., prior shape fitting, Markov-Gibbs random field) to optimize the binary segmentation accuracy. On the other end, [4] utilizes analytical shape and appearance priors and Markov-Gibbs random field; [1] designs elaborate region-growing criteria separating nodule growth from normal tissues; and [3] empowers morphological approaches and convexity models. CAD detection bias or dependency on segmentation (e.g., under- or over-segmentation often occurred, segmentation failures) may not be desirable as discussed in [5].

A Bayesian voxel labeling approach for lung nodule detection was thus proposed [5], avoiding explicit segmentation. Nevertheless, their four types of probabilistic formulations of nodule, vessel, vessel junction and outlier are based on medical literature description or general knowledge, but not verified from a large amount of data. For example, the nodule model is chosen as a solid ellipsoid with similar concentric ellipsoidal isosurfaces, and the vessel model represents a section of a solid torus with similar concentric isosurfaces. Their detailed model parameters are heuristically decided from common medical prior knowledge, for example, 15 mm for the average maximum radius of a pulmonary vessel. The nodule model in [5] is invalid for partial-solid and ground-glass nodules which nevertheless have great importance for CAD to perform well, as it is more ambiguous for radiologists. The solid parenchymal nodule model may also have trouble with other contextual types (e.g., juxta-pleural, pleural tail, and vascular [6]). The Bayesian closed-form mathematical representation of nodule, vessel, vessel junction, and outliers may be questionable whether the analytic models can describe well the tremendous anatomical appearance variations in hospital-size datasets. For example, the vessel junction is assumed to be a bifurcation structure in [5] whereas, from Fig. 1(d), the vascular anatomy describes four branches.

In this paper, we follow voxel classification framework [7,8], but our voxel-level labeling is data-driven and statistically learned from the annotated lesion image masks [6,9] on a number of CT scans. Only voxel probability assignment and thresholding (e.g., suppressing background clutter) are employed to obtain a lesion class-probability response map. Descriptive feature extraction based on instance-level spatial aggregation is then performed, without explicit segmentation optimization. Our system is trained using Bayesian multiple instance relevance vector machine (MILRVM) classifier [10] as a building-block through database-level selective training. The validation results of lung CAD on 879 CT scans collected from 10+ medical sites in US, Asia, Europe, are very promising. To the best of our knowledge, we are the first to report a unified, high-performance classification framework of detecting all solid, partial-solid, and ground-glass lung nodules, using the same set of supervisedly learned image features. This approach can be seamlessly applied to colonic polyp detection as well.

Our paper leverages discriminatively trained, higher-order image appearance model to label voxel class (e.g., polyp/nodule/vessel) probability map, with **mostly no segmentation level optimization**. Simple probability thresholding and connected component-based pruning are used. Then we extract a group of statistics or generative features in the dual space of learned probability and CT intensity volumes. These features are effective to fit our new hierarchical classification models, and yet flexible for different tasks. The proposed hierarchical feature learning approach is generic for identifying colon polyp, lung nodule, or vessel problems, in a unified and principled data-driven manner. We validate its effectiveness by evaluating the impacts on large-scale colon and lung CAD system performances (879 and 770 volumes respectively). The results are very encouraging and significantly outperform the recent state-of-the-arts [1,2,5,11–15].

2   Materials and Methods

Candidate Generation: CAD systems generally contain two stages: ROI (region of interest, or instance) candidate generation, and ROI feature learning & classification. Candidate generation (CG) is to rapidly identify anomalous regions with high sensitivity (e.g., >99 %) but low specificity, e.g. 150–200 candidates per scan, with typically zero to several true positives, in screening population. For convenience of comparison, we use the standard local shape index [16] method for extracting polyp candidates, and an efficient multiscale 3D Difference of Gaussians (DOG) filter to find potential nodule instances. In this paper, our focus is the later phase. The proposed method consists of voxel-level, instance-level, and database-level hierarchical feature learning, spatial aggregation, and final classification.

2.1   Supervised Probabilistic Voxel Map Labeling $\wp$ in ROI

Nodule, vessel, and polyp features were learned from 209, 56, and 427 training instances (i.e., voxel-annotated subvolumes in 3 dimensions of 41~83 voxels),

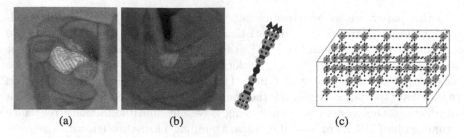

Fig. 2. (a,b) Examples of two polyps with annotated 3D contours and obtained probability map (brighter intensity indicates higher probability). Labeling noise is observed. (c) Steerable sampling grid patterns of labeling voxels on 3D surface (colon polyp) or in 3D volume (lung nodule and vessel) [19].

respectively. Examples are illustrated in Figs. 1 and 2. Training data represent a vast variety of lesions and vessels, with different intensity patterns, shape morphologies, adjacent contextual structures, and sizes (≥ 3 mm, highly correlated with actionability of a given lesion), as long as they are clinically relevant. CT images are isotropically resampled with the resolution of 1 mm. The training nodule or vessel instances are first cropped as subvolume ROI from the whole CT volume, based on ground-truth. Three clinical experts were asked to manually segment nodule and vessel using a "voxel-painting" tool where **Red** represents nodule and **Green** for vessel voxels. Polyp segmentation is defined as extracting the polyp surface area, via a closed 3D curve boundary on a colonic wall surface. A semi-automatic annotation tool was built for editing computer generated polyp segmentation contours, similar to [17]. The colon isosurface can be returned by running the Marching Cubes algorithm [18] to separate colon lumen from soft-tissue. After annotation, we obtained a set of labeled or masked voxels in each instance ROI for lesion or vessel. In total, there are 122215, 60335, or 190638 voxels to be treated as positive samples for training class probability of nodule, vessel, or polyp, respectively. Unmasked voxels located at least 3 mm away from labeled ones were initially treated as negatives, with resampling. The numbers of negative training samples are in general 4–6 times the sizes of positive sets.

Training and Features: We build the voxel-level classifier using probabilistic boosting tree (PBT[1]) training [20], coupled with 3D axis-sampled steerable features for polyp *surface voxels*, and 3D box-sampled feature patterns centered at nodule/vessel *volume voxels*. This step returns three classifiers $\{PBT_n; PBT_v; PBT_p\}$ for nodule/vessel/polyp, respectively. $\{PBT_n; PBT_v; PBT_p\}$ normally have 4–5 layers of internal nodes with 160–240 features selected. For details of image features for training of *surface voxels* and *volume voxels*, refer to [17,19].

---

[1] PBT is a powerful two-class and multiclass discriminative learning framework [20]. Random Forests or Ferns [21,22] are also applicable for training voxel-level labeler. Our empirical experience shows that PBT can learn very similar or slightly better ROC curves with much simpler model complexity, i.e., one tree versus multiple trees per model/classifier.

PBT training is assisted by cross-validation-based model selection on determining the tree depth. Note that the bootstrapping strategy on finding hard negative samples and retraining is not found particularly helpful.

Curvature features have demonstrated to be very helpful for parsing *surface voxels* [11,12,17], but appear not to provide much additional information gain on classifying *volume voxels*, especially in the case of nodule voxel detection. The other reason is that the previous work only focuses on solitary solid nodules [5,15] to show that curvature may be useful, whereas we train a single classifier PBT_n to handle all three types of nodules, under various anatomical contexts [6,23]. Partial solid and ground-glass can have very weak, noisy, and non-informative curvature features. Not computing Gaussian/principal curvatures in 3D volume space also improves the computational efficiency. The per-grid feature pool number drops from 71 to 23 for boosting feature selection.

Testing and Pruning: (1), In runtime testing, for each given 3D lesion candidate ROI obtained by a candidate generation process (which is common in CAD pipeline [3,12,17]), we exhaustively assign each ROI voxel v with its class probability value $\wp \in [0,1]$ by evaluating either one of $\{PBT_n; PBT_v; PBT_p\}$. Then we generate the label map for foreground (nodule, vessel, or polyp) voxels versus background ones, by simple thresholding on $\wp$-field: $L = 1$, if $\wp > \tau$; and $L = 0$, otherwise. From the training Receiver Operating Characteristic (ROC) performance of $\{PBT_n; PBT_v; PBT_p\}$, we can select the respective thresholds $\{\tau_n = 0.23; \tau_v = 0.45; \tau_p = 0.24\}$ to hold 98 % sensitivity. (2), Next, a fast connected component algorithm (26-neighborhood) is used to partition the L-field into separate clusters $\{C\}$. The cluster with the largest $\sum(\wp)$ from its support L map are kept (denoted as $\mathbb{S}$ where $L = 1$) and $L = 0$ is set for all remaining voxels, assuming there is only one dominating structure from each CAD candidate ROI. (3), After connected component base non-maximum pruning, we can effectively remove false positive responses while keeping high sensitivity. Based on our empirical evaluation, highly optimized segmentation procedures [6,11,17,24] may not improve the learned features with significantly better discriminativeness. For the detection purpose, our modeling of the voxel-level unary energy term (in a CRF sense) appears mostly sufficient. However the rough segmentation accuracy by detection is statistically lower than [17,24], e.g., for size measurement (tuned by τ towards over-segmentation for high detection sensitivity).

2.2 Spatial Aggregation Image Features (SAIF) in ROI

Voxels of different lesion types are mapped into the same universal $\wp$ space. Each voxel can be represented as a tuple of $(\wp, v, x_v, y_v, z_v)$ as probability, intensity, and spatial location. We compute the following SAIF feature groups per region of interest (ROI).

Statistics of Class Probability $\{\wp\}$ and Intensity $\{v\}$ (9): This feature group computes five overall statistics of $\{\wp\}$ in $\mathbb{S}$: $Prob_{Sum}$ is the sum of polyp-class posterior probabilities within segmentation $\sum\{\wp\}$; $Prob_{Avg}$ is the corresponding average probability $Prob_{Sum}/|\mathbb{S}|$, and its second to fourth order moments (i.e., standard deviation $Prob_{Std}$, skewness $Prob_{Skw}$ and kurtosis $Prob_{Kts}$). Similarly, we compute the $1st$–$4th$ order moments for the set of intensity distribution $\{v\}$.

3D Ellipsoid Shape Descriptor (10): For the 3D voxel mass $\mathbb{S}$ per ROI, we first estimate its centroid and covariance matrix in *volumetric* coordinates:

$$[\bar{x}, \bar{y}, \bar{z}] = \frac{\sum_{\mathbb{S}}[x_v, y_v, z_v] \times \wp}{\sum_{\mathbb{S}} \wp} \tag{1}$$

$$\text{CoMat} = \frac{\sum_{\mathbb{S}}(\Delta X)^T (\Delta X) \times \wp}{\sum_{\mathbb{S}} \wp} \tag{2}$$

where $\Delta X = [x_v, y_v, z_v] - [\bar{x}, \bar{y}, \bar{z}]$ Then, Singular Value Decomposition is used to calculate three Eigen-values of CoMat: R_1, R_2, R_3 that geometrically maps to the three radii if fitting the mass of $\mathbb{S}$ as an ellipsoid. The covariance matrix CoMat models the *3D volumetric spatial distribution* of underlying lesion or vessel confidence/probability in 3D CT images. Apart from standard Ellipsoid fitting, $\wp$ is used as a weight factor in Eqs. 1, 2, to reflect per-voxel class probability. Assuming $R_1 \geq R_2 \geq R_3$, six other features ($R_1 \times R_2 \times R_3$, $(R_1 \times R_2 \times R_3)^{1/3}$, $R_1 \times R_2, R_1/R_2, R_2/R_1, R_1/R_3, R_3/R_1$) are computed for feature expansion purpose. More sophisticated 3D shape features, such as "plateness", "stickness" and "ballness" [25], do not have superior performance than our ellipsoid based shape descriptor, from our empirical evaluation.

Multiscale Intensity Histogram Features (16): By using the $\wp$-weighted covariance matrix CoMat, we search all voxels $\{[v, x_v, y_v, z_v]\}$ within the $\sqrt{M}$ *Mahalanobis* distance, originating from the ellipsoid centroid $[\bar{x}, \bar{y}, \bar{z}]$, i.e.,

$$\text{MHD}(v) = (\Delta X)(\text{CoMat})^{-1}(\Delta X)^T \leq M \tag{3}$$

where $\Delta X = [x_v, y_v, z_v] - [\bar{x}, \bar{y}, \bar{z}]$. M is set as $2, 4, 6, 8$, corresponding to the fitted 3D object ellipsoids of multiple spatial scales and keeping their radii aspect ratios. A domain-knowledge based CT intensity binning of $[0, 350); [350, 950);$ $[950, 1100); [1100, 4095]$ is used to construct an intensity histogram $IH_k, k = 0, 1, 2, 3$ for each ellipsoid. Binning stands for air, soft tissue, fat and bone structures. Thus a total of 16 MIH features are calculated (4 bins by 4 scales) to model the intensity patterns in multiscale contexts. Deriving histograms in the image *Gradient* domain is also feasible [26] (left for future work).

Boundary Gradient-Shape Statistics Features (12): Given the $\wp$-thresholded voxel set (as a 3D point cloud) in the ROI, we first extract all boundary voxels $\{b\}$ with neighbors both inside and outside (i.e., $L = 1$ or 0). 26-neighborhood is used. The following three measurements are then computed.

$$NDist(b) = \|[x_b, y_b, z_b] - [\bar{x}, \bar{y}, \bar{z}]\| / D \tag{4}$$

$$NGrad(b) = \|\nabla(x_b, y_b, z_b)\| / G \tag{5}$$

$$Ori(b) = \frac{\nabla(x_b, y_b, z_b)}{\|\nabla(x_b, y_b, z_b)\|} \circ \frac{[x_b, y_b, z_b] - [\bar{x}, \bar{y}, \bar{z}]}{\|[x_b, y_b, z_b] - [\bar{x}, \bar{y}, \bar{z}]\|} \tag{6}$$

where D is the maximum of $\|[x_b, y_b, z_b] - [\bar{x}, \bar{y}, \bar{z}]\|$ in the boundary voxel set $\{b\}$; G is the maximum $\|\nabla(x_b, y_b, z_b)\|$ from training. Therefore distance $NDist(b)$ and gradient $NGrad(b)$ measurements are normalized $\in [0, 1]$ and scale-invariant. $Ori(b)$ is the dot-product ($\in [-1, +1]$) of the centroid-to-boundary direction and its local gradient direction which encodes boundary shape information. From $\{b\}$, we treat $\{NDist(b)\}$, $\{NGrad(b)\}$, $\{Ori(b)\}$ as three empirical distributions and compute their global statistics of $1st$–$4th$ order moments as features. These boundary gradient-shape features are related to 2D/3D ray features [27] describing irregular shapes, but more compact (without concatenating dozens of sampling directions) and truly rotation invariant for robustness.

Our spatially aggregated image features capture the joint intensity/shape and class-conditional probability $(\wp, \upsilon)$ statistics of all ROI voxels, which has not been explicitly addressed previously [1, 2, 5, 8, 12, 14]. These features model the high range/order spatial interactions among voxels within ROI, as an empirical distribution. Features are also translation and rotation invariant. **Most importantly, after Sect. 2.1, SAIF definition is universal for different types of lesions (e.g., polyp and nodule) and handle all their subtypes represented in training.**

2.3 Flexible Learning on Detection Using Soft Categorization

We design flexible tree-based classification hierarchies to optimize the final CAD detection performance, using image features computed for $(+/-)$ ROIs. Bayesian

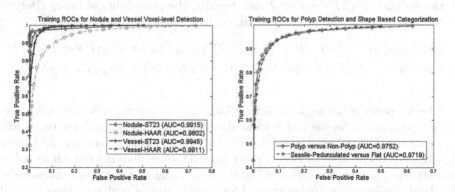

Fig. 3. ROC Curves of voxel-level learning: comparison of nodule and vessel voxel detection using 3D steerable features or Haar features with PBT training [20] **(Left)**; polyp versus non-polyp classification; Sessile-Pedunculated versus Flat polyp based shape categorization **(Right)**.

multiple instance relevance vector machine (MILRVM) [10] is adopted as the main building-block on classification of ROI features and soft-categorization. MILRVM is validated with good classification accuracy and generality, with feature selection and linear fusion.

Subcategory Soft-Gating: We propose a two-layer hierarchical classification architecture, called "soft-gating" framework in a Bayesian "divide-and-conquer" or mixture-of-experts setting. (1), A basic MILRVM [10] classifier is trained using *Sessile + Pedunculated* (SP) polyps versus *Flat* polyps in colon CAD; or *Wall-attached* (WA) versus *Nonwall-attached* (NWA) nodules in lung CAD, respectively. The main idea is that polyps under different shape morphologies present large within-class variations in feature space; nodules attached to a lung peripheral wall are expected to show different characteristics [6] when compared to isolated nodules. By handling these true positive lesion candidates separately according to the defined (sub)categorization, we can obtain a more robust classifier. Learning these category attributes may be partially informative for further lesion malignancy diagnosis. Similar Area-Under-Curve (AUC) measurements of ROC curves are obtained, by comparing polyp versus non-polyp voxel classification (AUC = 0.9752) or Sessile-Pedunculated versus Flat polyp categorization (AUC = 0.9719). (2), The leaf classifier is trained using the annotated lesions of the targeted category only (from ground-truth) versus all negatives. This binary tree classification framework is illustrated in Fig. 4(**Right**). Shallow tree is used here due to already hierarchically learned and strongly informative SAIF features and MILRVM.

In runtime, soft-gating means that all candidates will be passed into both left and right leaf classifiers to be evaluated, yet with a different category probability from the gating classifier (in contrast to hard-gating where candidates only run into either one of the tree branches.), such as $Pb(SP)$, $Pb(Flat)$, $Pb(W)$ and $Pb(NW)$. There is no need to normalize the pairs of weights (e.g., $Pb(SP) + Pb(Flat) = 1$) since we expect negative candidates to get low probabilities on both $Pb(SP)$ and $Pb(Flat)$. Finally, the probability of being "Polyp" or "Nodule" for any candidate is obtained in a Bayesian fusion manner:

$$Pb(Polyp) = Pb(SP) \times Pb_L(Polyp|SP) + Pb(Flat) \times Pb_R(Polyp|Flat) \quad (7)$$
$$Pb(Nodule) = Pb(W) \times Pb_L(Nodule|W) + Pb(NW) \times Pb_R(Nodule|NW)$$
$$(8)$$

The purposes of having a classifier which can distinguish different polyp categories (commonly Sessile and Pedunculated versus Flat polyps) are two folds: shape morphology labeling is helpful for radiologist decision making; and more importantly, it can help to have a good gate classifier dividing the whole polyp candidate population into different leaf branches, against their shape characteristics. Leaf classifiers are further trained for each branch. Combining the gate and leaf classifiers, a formed classification hierarchy with better classification accuracy and generality is normally expected, in the spirit of divide-and-conquer. Two schemes are performed and evaluated: (1) We break the positive pool of PBT_1 into two parts, according to the shape morphology labels of their rooting polyps as (Sessile and Pedunculated, +), or (Flat, -); then PBT_1^G is trained and its affiliated FPR features are used for the system Gate RVM classifier. (2) We enhance the negative training set of PBT_1^G by adding all negatives of PBT_1 for a new negative set (i.e., non-polyp voxels and flat polyp voxels). By keeping the positive training set of PBT_1^G, we train PBT_2^G which gets the generality of "gating FPR features" under control, against non-polyp voxels. Therefore, ideally only Sessile and Pedunculated polyps have high response; whereas flat polyps and polyp FPs receive low scores. An example is shown in Fig. 3.

Selective-Training False Positive Filter: The last stage of classification can be followed with an anatomy-based false positive (FP) filter classifier. We construct a new MILRVM classifier using all training nodules versus the most difficult FPs of vessels and vessel bifurcation or branches (Fig. 1(d)) in lung CAD. Denote that the lesion (+) probability from soft-gating is $Pb(+)^c$ and $Pb(+)^f$ for FP filter. We combine them in Eq. 2.3 and obtain the final $Pb(+)$ to be thresholded for free ROC analysis.

$$Pb(+) = 1 - (1 - Pb(+)^c)(1 - Pb(+)^f) \qquad (9)$$

For instance, a positive candidate with $Pb(+)^c = 0.8$ and $Pb(+)^f = 0.8$ will have final $Pb(+) = 1 - 0.2 \times 0.2 = 0.96$, while a confusing vessel FP of $Pb(+)^c = 0.8$ and $Pb(+)^f = 0.2$ gets $Pb(+) = 0.84$. We gain a new sizable classification margin $0.12 = 0.96 - 0.84$.

3 Experimental Results and Discussion

Data: We learn lung CAD image features and final classifiers based on 510 training CT cases with 717 solid nodules (SN), 124 partial solid nodules (PSN) and 91 ground-glass nodules (GGN), and evaluate the system performance on the validation dataset of 369 volumes including 462 SN, 93 PSN, and 51 GGN, respectively. In colon CAD, we have a total of 770 Tagged-prep CT scans with 239 polyps in the patient level and 416 polyps in the volume level for colon CAD study (120 patient-level or 226 volume-level polyps for validation. Each patient has two scans). Training and validation are split at patient level. Datasets were collected from 10+ hospitals from US, Europe and Asia. Various scanner vendors and screening imaging protocols are used. *We do not have access to datasets from other work that we compare here. However, given the diversified nature of data collection, our datasets are sufficiently representative for performance validation.*

Discriminative Feature Evaluation: We first study the performance of voxel-level supervised learning. For labeling nodule/vessel voxels, 3D Haar features are also feasible for PBT feature selection and boosting. However, Haar features do not apply to colonic surface voxel learning since it is not rotation-invariant and can be very memory and computationally expensive [28]. It is observed that 3D steerable features noticeably outperform 3D Haar features in learning nodule voxel classifier and perform comparably for classifying vessel voxels. Next, Fisher Discriminant Score (FDS) of any given SAIF image feature f is defined

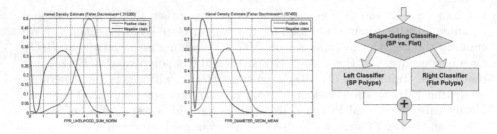

Fig. 4. Kernel Density Estimator plots of $Prob_{Sum}$ **(Left)** and Diameter_Geometry_Mean **(Middle)**, i.e., $(R_1 \times R_2 \times R_3)^{1/3}$, with the highest and $5th$ highest Fisher Discriminant (FD) scores of 1.3154 and 1.1575, respectively. **(Right:)** Shape Morphology based Soft-Gating Framework.

as $FD(f) = (\bar{f}^+ - \bar{f}^-)^2/(\sigma^2(f^+) + \sigma^2(f^-))$ where $\bar{f}^+$ and $\bar{f}^-$ denote the mean; $\sigma^2(f^+)$ and $\sigma^2(f^-)$ present the covariance of f distribution on positive $\{f^+\}$ and negative $\{f^-\}$ classes. FDS describes the gross two-class distribution separability or decision margin in a 1-dimensional feature space, as representing discriminativeness.

In Fig. 4, many SAIF features in Sect. 2.2 show excellent FD scores in polyp detection. The top three most informative feature groups are **Statistics of Voxel-Class Probability** $\{\wp\}$, **geometric dimensions from 3D Ellipsoid Shape Descriptor**, and surprisingly, **Boundary Gradient-Shape Statistics Features**. For example, the sum of probability feature $Prob_{Sum}$ and geometric mean diameter $(R_1 \times R_2 \times R_3)^{1/3}$ demonstrate excellent FD scores as 1.3154 and 1.1575 for single features. When size-gating is employed, boundary features show higher weights on the branch of large lesions which indicates more reliable feature computation as well. The supervisedly trained Probability features $\{\wp\}$ clearly outperform intensity feature groups. On the other hand, previous works employ and even heavily rely upon intensity information for detection and segmentation of lesions in CT images. In summary, $\{\wp\} >$ Gradient $>$ Intensity. Similar observations are also found for nodule SAIF features.

CAD Performance: Integrating our hierarchically learned SAIF image features into existing system for CAD training, achieves significantly higher detection rates under the same false positive (FP) rate and in terms of free ROCs (Fig. 5). In colon CAD validation dataset, with feature integrated, our shape-gated main classifier improves the per-patient actionable polyp detection sensitivity from 82.50 % [99/120] to 93.33 % [112/120], along with per-volume FP rate dropping to 2.18 from 2.85. Furthermore, it also improves the performance for detecting the relatively more difficult subcategory of flat polyps from 68.29 % [28/41] to 87.80 % [36/41], due to the "divide-and-conquer", SP versus flat polyp gating scheme. Six instance-level features based on SP versus Flat trained voxel labeler are selected with high weights for the gating MILRVM classifier of $Pb(SP)$, $Pb(Flat)$, out of 13 chosen features. Polyp features also strongly contribute to compose the left $Pb_L(Polyp|SP)$ and right $Pb_R(polyp|Flat)$ leaf classifiers.

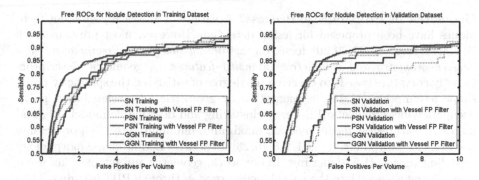

Fig. 5. Free ROC Curves of CAD system-level lung nodule detection in three categories: Solid Nodule (SN) in Blue; Partial Solid Nodule (PSN) in Red; and Ground-Glass Nodule (GGN) in Green, for both training (**Left**) and validation (**Right**) datasets. The impact of Vessel FP filter is evaluated (Color figure online).

For example, multiscale intensity histogram features help removing tagged stools and fatty polyps of no clinical significance, with higher intensity concentrations in outer bins. Spatial occupancy features eliminate tiny, spurious structures. As shown in Fig. 5 for both training and validation, the final wall versus non-wall gating + vessel FP filter consistently improves ROC performance for all three nodule categories and across datasets. Especially, harder-to-detect small solid nodules (3–4 mm) have higher sensitivity of 78.6 % [88/112] from 69.64 % [78/112]; and GGN of 84.3 % increased from 80.4 %. High sensitivities on detecting solid small and GGN nodules provide complementary and important values where radiologists may underperform, by employing CAD as a second reader. Using learned features with high FD scores helps the classifier generality from training to validation dataset.

Comparison: Our CAD performances compare favorably against the state-of-the-arts [1,2,5,8,12,14]. For Nodule detection, we achieve testing sensitivities of 90 % (SN ≥ 3 mm), 87.2 % (PSN), 84.3 % (GGN) and 78.6 % (small with 3–4 mm) at 4.1 FP/scan, while [2] reports sensitivity of 90.2 % at 8.2 FP/scan; [5] obtains 90 % sensitivity for non-calcified solid parenchymal nodules (≥4 mm) at 5.1 FP/Scan. Reference [8] manually preselects 140 CT volumes with at least one (≥4 mm) GGN nodule and reports sensitivity of 73 % at 1 FP/Scan (77–8 % at 4 FP/Scan) for GGN nodule detection only. For comparison on dataset scales, [5] uses 60 nodules from 50 CT scans under a single imaging protocol. Reference [2] employs 108 thoracic CT scans using a wide range of tube dose levels which contain 220 nodules (185 solid and 35 GGN). We report results on total 879 volumes of 1179 solid, 217 partial solid and 142 ground-glass nodules, which is the largest. For Polyp detection, our testing sensitivities are 93.3 % (SP≥ 3 mm) and 87.8 % (Flat) at 2.18 FP/scan, while [12] achieves 85–95 % (SP ≥ 6 mm) sensitivities at 5 FP/scan. Reference [14] reports 90 % (SP ≥ 6 mm) and 75–80 % (flat) at 4.5 FP/scan. In colon CAD, we use 770 Tagged-prep CT scans of multiple sites, among the largest studies with [12,14].

Geometric or Probabilistic Process? A variety of drastically different techniques have been proposed for lesion detection. However, most previous work [1, 2, 5, 11, 12, 15, 16, 23, 29, 30] focus on *extracting low-level, directly observable surface geometry and volumetric intensity features*: as geometric descriptors (mostly curvature based) to describe the degree of satisfying the sphericity polyp shape assumption [11, 16], segmentation or geometric protrusion based polyp occupancy measurements [12], fuzzy clustering and deformable model [29], and intensity features (as mean, median, maximum, minimum, etc.) [30] or Hessian statistics for polyp detection. [1, 2, 5, 15, 23] all address nodule shape morphology modeling versus other structures. In our work, geometry and intensity information are first encoded into the voxel labeling process through PBT learning. Then translation and rotation invariant visual features are computed summarizing the joint distribution of intensity and learned lesion-class probability.

Is Data-driven Learning Required for Large Data? Probabilistic approach of modeling the shape differences between polyps and other colonic surface structures is exploited [13] in a Bayesian closed-form mathematical formulation. Similarly, [5] discusses its counterpart in nodule detection. Both work derive features based on the shape, intensity prior knowledge presented in the medical literature. From a large scale annotated polyp/nodule segmentation dataset (e.g., hundreds of volumes and lesions), their analytic models do not fit well the huge anatomical appearance variation. Our voxel-level labeling is data-driven and supervisedly learned from annotated object image masks [6, 9, 17] on vast datasets (for better image generality). Consequently, [5, 13] report significantly inferior performance results on very limited datasets of 36 volumes and 24 polyps and 50 volumes with 60 solitary solid nodules. Apart from another learning based 3D polyp detection approach [28], our learning and parsing processes are efficiently performed on the colonic surface rather than exhaustively searching in subvolumes. Therefore the difficulty of detecting variable-posed 3D volumetric objects is completely avoided, while the required sample alignment in [28] by rotating 3D volumes is very time-consuming.

4   Conclusion

Our main contributions are four-fold. First, a flexible, hierarchical feature learning framework is presented, integrating different levels (voxel-, ROI instance- and database-level) of discriminative and descriptive information for CAD. Second, we propose Spatial Aggregation Image Features (insensitive to segmentation noises) to encode the robust statistics from voxel labeling responses within each ROI. Third, our approach provides a unified solution of detecting all types of nodules (solid, partial-solid, ground-glass) and polyps (sessile, pedunculated, flat; large, small), via the learned image features. Image appearance of different lesion categories are mapped into the universal $\wp$-probability space whereas previous work design different methods for each lesion type [5, 8, 12]. Last, we validate CAD performances on large-scale datasets achieving comparable or higher sensitivity at significantly lower FP rates, against the state-of-the-arts [1, 2, 5, 8, 12].

References

1. Dehmeshki, J., Amin, H., Valdivieso, M., Ye, X.: Segmentation of pulmonary nodules in thoracic CT scans: a region growing approach. IEEE Trans. Med. Imag. **27**, 467–480 (2008)
2. Ye, X., Lin, X., Dehmeshki, J., Slabaugh, G., Beddoe, G.: Shape based computer-aided detection of lung nodules in thoracic CT images. IEEE Trans. Biomed. Eng. **56**(7), 1810–1820 (2009)
3. Kubota, T., Jerebko, A., Dewan, M., Salganicoff, M., Krishnan, A.: Segmentation of pulmonary nodules of various densities with morphological approaches and convexity models. Med. Image Anal. **15**(1), 133–154 (2011)
4. El-Baz, A., Gimel'farb, G.: Robust medical images segmentation using learned shape and appearance models. In: Yang, G.-Z., Hawkes, D., Rueckert, D., Noble, A., Taylor, C. (eds.) MICCAI 2009, Part I. LNCS, vol. 5761, pp. 281–288. Springer, Heidelberg (2009)
5. Mendonça, P.R.S., Bhotika, R., Zhao, F., Miller, J.V.: Lung nodule detection via bayesian voxel labeling. In: Karssemeijer, N., Lelieveldt, B. (eds.) IPMI 2007. LNCS, vol. 4584, pp. 134–146. Springer, Heidelberg (2007)
6. Wu, D., Lu, L., Bi, J., Shinagawa, Y., Boyer, K., Krishnan, A., Salganicoff, M.: Stratified learning of local anatomical context for lung nodules in CT images. In: IEEE CVPR (2010)
7. Lo, P., Sporring, J., Ashraf, H., Pedersen, J., de Bruijne, M.: Vessel-guided airway tree segmentation: a voxel classification approach. Med. Image Anal. **14**, 527–538 (2010)
8. Jacobs, C., Sánchez, C.I., Saur, S.C., Twellmann, T., de Jong, P.A., van Ginneken, B.: Computer-aided detection of ground glass nodules in thoracic CT images using shape, intensity and context features. In: Fichtinger, G., Martel, A., Peters, T. (eds.) MICCAI 2011, Part III. LNCS, vol. 6893, pp. 207–214. Springer, Heidelberg (2011)
9. Shotton, J., Winn, J., Rother, C., Criminisi, A.: Textonboost for image understanding: multi-class object recognition and segmentation by jointly modeling texture, layout, and context. IJCV **81**(1), 1:2–1:23 (2009)
10. Raykar, V., Krishnapuram, B., Bi, J., Dundar, M., Rao, R.: Bayesian multiple instance learning: automatic feature selection and inductive transfer. In: ICML, pp. 808–815 (2008)
11. Jerebko, A.K., Lakare, S., Cathier, P., Periaswamy, S., Bogoni, L.: Symmetric curvature patterns for colonic polyp detection. In: Larsen, R., Nielsen, M., Sporring, J. (eds.) MICCAI 2006. LNCS, vol. 4191, pp. 169–176. Springer, Heidelberg (2006)
12. van Wijk, C., van Ravesteijn, V., Vos, F., van Vliet, L.J.: Detection and segmentation of colonic polyps on implicit isosurfaces by second principal curvature flow. IEEE Trans. Med. Imag. **29**(3), 688–698 (2010)
13. Melonakos, J., Mendonça, P.R.S., Bhotka, R., Sirohey, S.A.: A probabilistic model for haustral curvatures with applications to colon CAD. In: Ayache, N., Ourselin, S., Maeder, A. (eds.) MICCAI 2007, Part II. LNCS, vol. 4792, pp. 420–427. Springer, Heidelberg (2007)
14. Slabaugh, G., Yang, X., Ye, X., Boyes, R., Beddoe, G.: A robust and fast system for ctc computer-aided detection of colorectal lesions. Algorithms **3**(1), 21–43 (2010)
15. Mendonça, P.R.S., Bhotika, R., Sirohey, S.A., Turner, W.D., Miller, J.V., Avila, R.S.: Model-based analysis of local shape for lesion detection in CT scans. In: Duncan, J.S., Gerig, G. (eds.) MICCAI 2005. LNCS, vol. 3749, pp. 688–695. Springer, Heidelberg (2005)

16. Paik, D., et al.: Surface normal overlap: a computer-aided detection algorithm with application to colonic polyps and lung nodules in helical CT. IEEE Trans. Med. Imag. **23**(6), 661–675 (2004)
17. Lu, L., Barbu, A., Wolf, M., Liang, J., Bogoni, L., Salganicoff, M., Comaniciu, D.: Accurate polyp segmentation for 3D CT colonography using multi-staged probabilistic binary learning and compositional model. In: IEEE CVPR (2008)
18. Lorensen, W., Cline, H.: Marching cubes: a high resolution 3D surface construction algorithm. ACM SIGGRAPH Comput. Graph. **21**(4), 163–169 (1987)
19. Lu, L., Barbu, A., Wolf, M., Liang, J., Bogoni, L., Salganicoff, M., Comaniciu, D.: Simultaneous detection and registration for ileo-cecal valve detection in 3D CT colonography. In: European Conference on Computer Vision, vol. 4, pp. 10–15 (2008)
20. Tu, Z.: Probabilistic boosting-tree: Learning discriminative models for classification, recognition, and clustering. In: ICCV, pp. 1589–1596 (2005)
21. Bosch, A., Zisserman, A., Munoz, X.: Image classification using random forests and ferns. In: ICCV, pp. 1–8 (2007)
22. Schwing, A., Zach, C., Zheng, Y., Pollefeys, M.: Adaptive random forest-how many experts to ask before making a decision? In: CVPR, pp. 1377–1384 (2011)
23. Farag, A., Graham, J., Farag, A., Falk, R.: Lung nodule modeling - a data-driven approach. In: Bebis, G. (ed.) ISVC 2009. LNCS, vol. 5875, pp. 347–356. Springer, Heidelberg (2009)
24. Lu, L., Bi, J., Wolf, M., Salganicoff, M.: Effective 3D object detection and regression using probabilistic segmentation features in CT images. In: IEEE Computer Vision and Pattern Recognition, pp. 1–8 (2011)
25. Gorelick, L., Blank, M., Shechtman, E., Irani, M., Basri, R.: Actions as space-time shapes. IEEE Trans. Pattern Anal. Mach. Intell. **29**, 2247–2253 (2007)
26. Toews, M., Wells, W.M.: Efficient and robust model-to-image alignment using 3D scale-invariant features. Med. Image Anal. **17**(3), 271–282 (2013)
27. Smith, K., Carleton, A., Lepetit, V.: Fast ray features for learning irregular shapes. In: ICCV (2009)
28. Tu, Z., Zhou, X., Bogoni, L., Barbu, A., Comaniciu, D.: Probabilistic 3D polyp detection in CT images: the role of sample alignment. In: CVPR, pp. 1544–1551 (2006)
29. Yao, J., Miller, M., Franaszek, M., Summers, R.: Colonic polyp segmentation in CT colongraphy-based on fuzzy clustering and deformable models. IEEE Trans. Med. Imag. **23**(11), 1344–1352 (2004)
30. van Ravesteijn, V., van Wijk, C., Vos, F., Truyen, R., Peters, J., Stoker, J., van Vliet, L.: Computer aided detection of polyps in CT colonography using logistic regression. IEEE Trans. Med. Imag. **29**(11), 1907–1917 (2010)

Shape Curvature Histogram: A Shape Feature for Celiac Disease Diagnosis

Michael Gadermayr[1(✉)], Michael Liedlgruber[1], Andreas Uhl[1], and Andreas Vécsei[2]

[1] Department of Computer Sciences, University of Salzburg, Salzburg, Austria
{mgadermayr,mliedl,uhl}@cosy.sbg.ac.at
http://www.wavelab.at
[2] Endoscopy Unit, St. Anna Children's Hospital, Vienna, Austria

Abstract. In this work we introduce a curvature based shape feature extraction technique. To construct the proposed descriptor, first an input color channel is subject to edge detection and gradient computations. Then, based on the gradient map and edge map, the local curvature of the contour is computed for each pixel as the angular difference between the maximum and minimum gradient angle within a certain neighborhood. Experiments show, that the feature is competitive as far as the classification rate is concerned. Despite its discriminative power, a further positive aspect is the compactness of the feature vector.

1 Introduction

Celiac disease is a complex autoimmune disorder in genetically predisposed individuals of all age groups after introduction of gluten containing food. The real prevalence of the disease has not been fully clarified yet. This is due to the fact that most patients with celiac disease suffer from no or atypical symptoms and only a minority develops the classical form of the disease. Since several years, prevalence data have been continuously adjusted upwards. Fasano et al. state that more than 2 million people in the United States, this is about one in 133, have the disease [1]. Endoscopy with biopsy is currently considered the gold standard for the diagnosis of celiac disease. Due to the technological advances in endoscopy throughout the past years, modern endoscopes also allow to capture images, which facilitates automated analysis and diagnosis. Thus, automated classification as a support tool is an emerging option for endoscopic diagnosis and treatments [2].

In the past various different approaches for an automated classification of celiac disease images have been proposed. The majority of these approaches investigated different texture features for the classification. Features utilized throughout these works include for example simple statistical features [3], statistical features on color histograms [4] and statistical features extracted from Fourier magnitudes [5]. In the studies presented in [6,7] an extensive comparison between various different types of features (e.g. wavelet-based, Fourier-based,

B. Menze et al. (Eds.): MCV 2013, LNCS 8331, pp. 175–184, 2014.
DOI: 10.1007/978-3-319-05530-5_17, © Springer International Publishing Switzerland 2014

Random fields, and Local Binary Pattern variants) has been conducted. In [7] two shape-based approaches have been evaluated [8,9], which – to the best of our knowledge – are the only two shape-based approaches ever evaluated for an automated diagnosis of celiac disease. Actually, there exists different definitions of shape-based features. We define a feature to be shape-based, if it is based on previously detected edges or one or more segmented objects.

Compared to the results obtained with the texture features the shape-based method proposed in [8] yielded rather poor results only. The main cause for this is the fact that the feature used in this work has been specifically tailored to another problem domain (i.e. measures the pit density on colonic polyps for a classification). The second shape-based method (from [9]), is based on feature subset selection. The pool of possible features for subset selection included various different shape features (e.g. perimeter or area of closed regions found). This method performed rather well in terms of the classification rates achieved.

In this work we present a novel shape-based feature, called Shape Curvature Histogram (SCH). This feature describes the curvature of shapes found within an image in the form of a compact histogram. In contrast to many other shape-based features the SCH feature does not require shapes with closed boundaries which could be difficult or even impossible to obtain if single objects cannot be identified. Thereby our approach is a very general one and can potentially be applied to other problem domains as well.

The remaining part of this paper is organized as follows: In Sect. 2, our new feature extraction approach is explained. In Sect. 3, experimental results imply a high discriminative power with a compact feature representation. Section 4 concludes this paper.

2   Shape Curvature Histogram (SCH)

The computation of the SCH feature can be divided into the following steps: edge map generation, orientation computation, curvature computation, and the creation of the final feature vector.

In the explanations below I denotes the image the SCH feature should be computed for. If I is a grayscale image the computation steps are carried out only once, resulting in a single histogram. For RGB images the steps are carried out for each color channel separately, resulting in one histogram for each color channel. These histograms are then concatenated in order to obtain the final feature vector.

In the following we explain the computation steps in more detail. For details on the implementation, we refer to the provided MATLAB reference implementation.[1] The average execution runtime for a 128×128 pixel gray value image on an Intel i5 (3.1 GHz) architecture is 0.012 s.

---

[1] The MATLAB reference implementation can be downloaded from http://www.wavelab.at/sources/Gadermayr12f.

2.1   Edge Map Generation

To be able to compute the curvature information the first step is the generation of an edge map. For this purpose we employ the Canny edge detector [10]. The result of the edge detection is an edge map which contains all pixels for which we compute the curvature values. In other words, pixels which do not belong to an edge are masked out from the computation steps below. Although in special cases the edge map might contain closed boundaries, generally the edge map could consist of an arbitrary number of disconnected parts of arbitrary shapes. Thus, we can not make any assumption on the existence of closed boundaries, which would be obligatory for contour-based or region-based shape feature extraction techniques.

2.2   Computation of Orientation

Once the edge map is generated, we compute the gradient direction for each edge pixel. Having both partial derivatives, this direction can be calculated as[2]

$$\Theta(x, y) = \text{atan2} \left(\frac{\partial I}{\partial y}(x, y), \frac{\partial I}{\partial x}(x, y) \right) , \quad (1)$$

where (x, y) denotes the position of the edge pixel for which the orientation is computed. The resulting values for $\Theta(x, y)$ always lie within the range $(-\pi, \pi)$.

The partial derivatives $\frac{\partial I}{\partial x}$ and $\frac{\partial I}{\partial y}$ are approximated by a convolution of the image with Sobel filters. Figure 1(e) shows an example orientation image, which has been computed from the example image shown in Fig. 1(a) and the edge map shown in Fig. 1(b).

2.3   Computation of Curvature

Having the orientation for each edge pixel, we compute the curvature for an edge pixel as the difference between the maximum and minimum gradient angle over all edge pixels within a certain neighborhood. The curvature C for an edge pixel located at (x, y) can thus be formulated as:

$$C(x, y) = D(\Theta_{\min}(x, y), \Theta_{\max}(x, y)) , \quad (2)$$

with

$$\Theta_{\min}(x, y) = \min_{(i,j) \in N(x,y)} \Theta(i, j) \quad (3)$$

and

$$\Theta_{\max}(x, y) = \max_{(i,j) \in N(x,y)} \Theta(i, j) , \quad (4)$$

where $N(x, y)$ denotes the set of pixel positions of edge pixels within an $w \times w$-neighborhood centered at (x, y) (w denotes the width and height of the neighborhood). The difference between two arbitrary gradient directions might yield

---

[2] The function atan2 denotes the four-quadrant implementation of the atan-function.

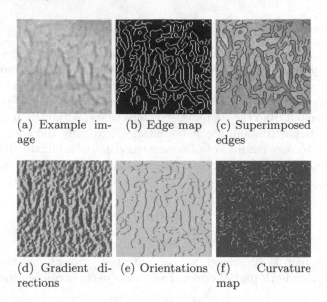

(a) Example im-   (b) Edge map   (c) Superimposed
age   edges

(d) Gradient di-   (e) Orientations   (f)   Curvature
rections   map

Fig. 1. Output of the different steps when extracting the SCH feature for a grayscale image. (a) the input image, (b) the corresponding edge map, (c) the edge map superimposed to the input image, (d) the gradient directions for the input image, (e) the edge pixel orientations (gradient directions, masked by the edge map), and (f) the final image showing the curvature values for the edge pixels (based on a 3×3-neighborhood).

two different types of angles: either an angle in the range $[0, \pi]$ or the respective reflex angle in the range $(\pi, 2\pi)$. Since we are only interested in angle differences in the range $[0, \pi]$, we quite often need to compute the smaller angle from the reflex angle. Hence, we use the following formula to compute the difference between two angles α and β:

$$D(\alpha, \beta) = \begin{cases} \Delta(\alpha, \beta), & \text{if } \Delta(\alpha, \beta) \leq \pi, \\ 2\pi - \Delta(\alpha, \beta), & \text{if } \Delta(\alpha, \beta) > \pi \end{cases}, \tag{5}$$

$$\Delta(\alpha, \beta) = \max(\alpha, \beta) - \min(\alpha, \beta). \tag{6}$$

A schematic illustration of the pixel-wise curvature computation is provided in Fig. 2. Figure 1(f) shows an example for a curvature map based on the input image shown in Fig. 1(a). In this figure different curvature values are represented by different colors.

2.4   Generation of Feature Vector

Based on the curvature values for the edge pixels a histogram is created. For the construction of a histogram we do not consider curvature values of non-edge pixels since these contain no information anyway (due to the restriction of the curvature computation to edge pixels). Hence, the number of pixels contributing

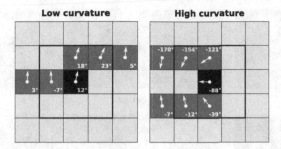

Fig. 2. Computation of the curvature for a pixel (black, filled square). The gradient directions for the edge pixels (shown in dark gray) are indicated by arrows (the according angles are given in degrees). The 3×3-neighborhood used in this example is indicated by a black square. While the left image shows an example for a low curvature value ($C(x,y) = 30°$), the right image shows a rather high curvature ($C(x,y) = 142°$).

to the curvature histogram is likely to change from image to image. As a consequence we normalize each histogram by the number of edge pixels found in the respective image.

The limits of the histograms cover the complete range of possible curvature values (i.e. $[0, \pi]$). The number of bins to be used for histogram creation can be adjusted. The higher the number of bins the more detailed the curvature values get captured by the resulting histogram. But the length of the resulting feature vectors will also be higher. In addition, in case of too many bins the bin values may get rather noisy, making the feature unstable in terms of the classification. If, in contrast, the number of bins is too low, potentially discriminative information may get lost in the histogram, with the advantage of a more compact descriptor.

In our experiments we use 8 bins for our histograms, which yields high classification results although the feature vectors are compact. We did not achieve higher accuracies with a higher number of bins. The choice for the number of bins corresponds to a range of $\pi/8$ (i.e. 22.5°) covered by each bin.

3   Experiments

3.1   Experimental Setup

The image database used throughout our experiments is based on images taken during duodenoscopies at the St. Anna Children's Hospital, using pediatric gastroscopes without magnification (GIF-Q165 and GIF-N180, Olympus).

The main indications for endoscopy were the diagnostic evaluation of dyspeptic symptoms, positive celiac serology, anemia, malabsorption syndromes, inflammatory bowel disease, and gastrointestinal bleeding. Images were recorded by using the modified immersion technique, which is based on the instillation of water into the duodenal lumen for better visibility of the villi. Using this technique, the tip of the gastroscope is inserted into the water and images of interesting areas are taken. A study [11] shows that the visualization of villi

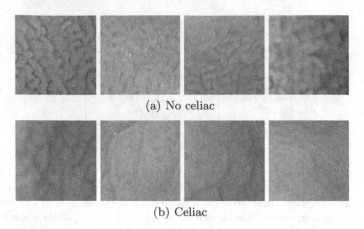

(a) No celiac

(b) Celiac

Fig. 3. Patches of patients without (a) and with the disease (b).

with the immersion technique has a higher positive predictive value. Previous work [6] also found that the modified immersion technique is more suitable for automated classification purposes as compared to the classical image capturing technique (Fig. 3).

To study the prediction accuracy of different features we manually created an "idealistic" set of textured image patches with optimal quality. Thus, the data was inspected and filtered by several qualitative factors (sharpness, distortions, and visibility of features). In the next step, patches with a fixed size of 128×128 pixels were extracted (a size which turned out to be optimally suited in earlier experiments on automated celiac disease diagnosis [6]). This way we created an extended set containing more images available for classification. In order to generate ground truth for the texture patches used in experimentation, the condition of the mucosal areas covered by the images was determined by histological examination of biopsies from the corresponding regions.

Table 1 shows the detailed ground truth information used for our experiments where N_O, N_E, N_P denote the number of original images, the number of extracted (idealistic) image patches used for classification, and the number of patients in each class, respectively.

To estimate the classification accuracy of our system we use leave-one-patient-out cross-validation (LOPO-CV). In this setup one image out of the database

Table 1. The detailed ground truth information for the celiac disease image database used throughout our experiments.

	N_O	N_E	N_P
No celiac	234	306	131
Celiac	172	306	40
Total	**406**	**612**	**171**

is considered as an unknown image. The remaining images are used to train the classifier (omitting those images which originate from the same patient as the image left out). To actually classify an unknown image (not contained in the training set) we use the k-nearest-neighbor classifier (k-NN). This rather simple classifier has been chosen to emphasize more on quantifying the discriminative power of the features proposed in this work.

To measure the distance between two histograms we employ the histogram intersection distance metric. We also carried out experiments using other distance metrics (the Euclidean distance metric and the Bhattacharyya distance metric) but the classification results were rather similar to those obtained with the histogram intersection distance metric.

Since the optimal choices for the k-value for the k-NN classifier are not known beforehand, we decided to carry out an exhaustive search for the k-value which leads to the highest overall classification rates ($k \in 1, \ldots, 50$). Apart from that we carry out experiments with grayscale images as well as with RGB color images. In case of RGB images, a feature vector is extracted for each color channel. These are then concatenated to end up with the final feature vector. In order to compute the local curvature values (see Eq. (2)), we used a 3×3-neighborhood. While bigger neighborhoods are theoretically possible, experiments showed that, especially in case of dense edge maps (i.e. a high number of edge pixels), bigger neighborhoods are more likely to interfere with edge pixels from different edges.

We also aim at a comparison between the proposed method and a set of four features proposed in the past. These features include texture-based features as well as shape-based features:

- **Graylevel Co-occurrence Matrix features (GLCM)** [12]
  The GLCM is a 2D-histogram, which describes the spatial relationship between neighboring pixels. To obtain features for the classification, a GLCM for four different directions (and offset 1 pixel) is computed. Then a subset of the statistical features proposed in [12] (i.e. contrast, correlation, energy, and homogeneity) on each GLCM is extracted. The final features used are composed by concatenating the Haralick features.
- **Edge Co-occurrence Matrix (ECM)** [13]
  After applying eight differently orientated directional filters, the orientation (maximal response) is determined for each pixel, followed by masking out pixels with a gradient magnitude below some threshold (75 % below the maximum response in our experiments). Then the methodology of GLCM is used to obtain the ECM for one specific displacement (1 pixel displacement in our experiments).
- **Local Binary Patterns (LBP)** [14]
  The well known LBP are utilized in its common configuration with 8 circularly arranged neighbors and a radius of 1 pixel.
- **Shape features combination (EDGEFEATURES)** [9]
  After Canny Edge detection, different features from edge-enclosed regions are computed. In the original paper [9] edge shape features and texture features were used. However, for the results in this work we use shape features only.

To find the most discriminative combination of features we use a greedy forward feature subset selection.

In order to be able to assess whether two different methods produce statistically significant differences in the results obtained, we employ McNemar's test [15] (with a significance level of $\alpha = 0.05$).

3.2 Results

Table 2 shows the detailed results for our experiments. The column "SD" in this table indicates whether there is a statistically significant difference between the results obtained with the SCH method and the other methods according to McNemar's test. In addition, the sign given in brackets indicates whether the results obtained are significantly lower ($-$) or significantly higher ($+$) as compared to the results of the SCH method. The last column (SCS) provides the information whether there is a statistically significant difference between the results for a specific method when comparing the grayscale and color results.

From these results we immediately notice that the SCH feature yields the highest overall classification rate (accuracy) as compared to the other features. This accounts to the results with grayscale images as well as to the color images results. We also notice that SCH in most cases delivers significantly higher results when compared to the other methods. Only in case of LBP applied to the grayscale images the difference to SCH is not significant, although also in this case SCH delivers a higher classification accuracy.

We also see that there are two methods only, which deliver a slightly higher accuracy when extracting the features from color images (i.e. GLCM and EDGE-FEATURES). In case of all other methods we observe a slight decrease of the accuracy in case of color images. But, except for the LBP method, the differences observed are not significantly different.

Table 2. Detailed classification rates obtained for grayscale images and color images.

Grayscale Images Method	Accuracy	Specificity	Sensitivity	SD	SCS
SCH	87.58	89.87	85.29		
ECM	77.45	75.16	79.74	✓ ($-$)	
GLCM	73.69	67.97	79.41	✓ ($-$)	
LBP	84.97	82.35	87.58		✓ ($-$)
EDGEFEATURES	67.16	75.49	58.82	✓ ($-$)	
RGB Color Images Method	Accuracy	Specificity	Sensitivity	SD	SCS
SCH	85.78	89.22	82.35		
ECM	76.31	78.10	74.51	✓ ($-$)	
GLCM	75.98	74.84	77.12	✓ ($-$)	
LBP	81.54	80.72	82.35	✓ ($-$)	✓ ($+$)
EDGEFEATURES	70.92	75.82	66.01	✓ ($-$)	

When looking at the results yielded by the EDGEFEATURES method we notice that the results are considerably lower as compared to the SCH method. This is especially interesting since the EDGEFEATURES method employs a feature selection algorithm, which – at least theoretically – should be advantageous.

4   Conclusion

We proposed a novel shape-based feature which we successfully applied to the problem of automated celiac disease diagnosis. We showed that, although the descriptor used is very compact, we in most cases achieve significantly higher classification accuracies as compared to some well-established feature extraction methods (texture features as well as shape-based features). We also showed that the SCH method can be easily extended to work with RGB color images. However, compared to the accuracy in case of grayscale images, the accuracy changes observed in our experiments are not statistically significant. Since the proposed feature has not been tailored specifically to celiac disease images (i.e. it makes no assumptions about the edges and gradients used), it may be potentially applied to other problem domains as well.

Acknowledgment. This work is partially funded by the Austrian Science Fund (FWF) under Project No. 24366.

References

1. Fasano, A., Berti, I., Gerarduzzi, T., Not, T., Colletti, R.B., Drago, S., Elitsur, Y., Green, P.H.R., Guandalini, S., Hill, I.D., Pietzak, M., Ventura, A., Thorpe, M., Kryszak, D., Fornaroli, F., Wasserman, S.S., Murray, J.A., Horvath, K.: Prevalence of celiac disease in at-risk and not-at-risk groups in the united states: a large multicenter study. Arch. Intern. Med. **163**, 286–292 (2003)
2. Liedlgruber, M., Uhl, A.: Computer-aided decision support systems for endoscopy in the gastrointestinal tract: a review. IEEE Rev. Biomed. Eng. **4**, 73–88 (2012)
3. Ciaccio, E.J., Tennyson, C.A., Lewis, S.K., Krishnareddy, S., Bhagat, G., Green, P.H.: Distinguishing patients with celiac disease by quantitative analysis of video capsule endoscopy images. Comput. Methods Programs Biomed. **100**(1), 39–48 (2010)
4. Vécsei, A., Fuhrmann, T., Uhl, A.: Towards automated diagnosis of celiac disease by computer-assisted classification of duodenal imagery. In: Proceedings of the 4th International Conference on Advances in Medical, Signal and Information Processing (MEDSIP '08), Santa Margherita Ligure, Italy, pp. 1–4, paper no P2.1-009 (2008)
5. Vécsei, A., Fuhrmann, T., Liedlgruber, M., Brunauer, L., Payer, H., Uhl, A.: Automated classification of duodenal imagery in celiac disease using evolved fourier feature vectors. Comput. Methods Programs Biomed. **95**, S68–S78 (2009)
6. Hegenbart, S., Kwitt, R., Liedlgruber, M., Uhl, A., Vécsei, A.: Impact of duodenal image capturing techniques and duodenal regions on the performance of automated diagnosis of celiac disease. In: Proceedings of the 6th International Symposium on Image and Signal Processing and Analysis (ISPA '09), Salzburg, Austria, September 2009, pp. 718–723 (2009)

7. Gschwandtner, M., Liedlgruber, M., Uhl, A., Vécsei, A.: Experimental study on the impact of endoscope distortion correction on computer-assisted celiac disease diagnosis. In: Proceedings of the 10th International Conference on Information Technology and Applications in Biomedicine (ITAB'10), Corfu, Greece, November 2010 (2010)

8. Häfner, M., Gangl, A., Liedlgruber, M., Uhl, A., Vécsei, A., Wrba, F.: Classification of endoscopic images using delaunay triangulation-based edge features. In: Campilho, A., Kamel, M. (eds.) ICIAR 2010, Part II. LNCS, vol. 6112, pp. 131–140. Springer, Heidelberg (2010)

9. Häfner, M., Gangl, A., Liedlgruber, M., Uhl, A., Vécsei, A., Wrba, F.: Endoscopic image classification using edge-based features. In: Proceedings of the 20th International Conference on Pattern Recognition (ICPR'10), Istanbul, Turkey, August 2010, pp. 2724–2727 (2010)

10. Canny, J.: A computational approach to edge detection. IEEE Trans. Pattern Recogn. Mach. Intell. **8**(6), 679–698 (1986)

11. Gasbarrini, A., Ojetti, V., Cuoco, L., Cammarota, G., Migneco, A., Armuzzi, A., Pola, P., Gasbarrini, G.: Lack of endoscopic visualization of intestinal villi with the immersion technique in overt atrophic celiac disease. Gastrointest. Endosc. **57**, 348–351 (2003)

12. Haralick, R.M., Shanmugam, K., Dinstein, I.: Textural features for image classification. IEEE Trans. Syst. Man Cybern. **3**, 610–621 (1973)

13. Rautkorpi, R., Iivarinen, J.: A novel shape feature for image classification and retrieval. In: Campilho, A., Kamel, M.S. (eds.) ICIAR 2004. LNCS, vol. 3211, pp. 753–760. Springer, Heidelberg (2004)

14. Ojala, T., Pietikäinen, M., Harwood, D.: A comparative study of texture measures with classification based on feature distributions. Pattern Recogn. **29**(1), 51–59 (1996)

15. Everitt, B.: The Analysis of Contingency Tables. Chapman and Hall, London (1977)

2D–Based 3D Volume Retrieval Using Singular Value Decomposition of Detected Regions

Alba García Seco de Herrera[1]([✉]), Antonio Foncubierta–Rodríguez[1],
Emanuele Schiavi[2], and Henning Müller[1]

[1] University of Applied Sciences Western Switzerland (HES–SO),
Sierre, Switzerland
alba.garcia@hevs.ch
[2] University Rey Juan Carlos, Madrid, Spain

Abstract. In this paper, a novel 3D retrieval model to retrieve medical volumes using 2D images as input is proposed. The main idea consists of applying a multi–scale detection of saliency of image regions. Then, the 3D volumes with the regions for each of the scales are associated with a set of projections onto the three canonical planes. The 3D shape is indirectly represented by a 2D–shape descriptor so that the 3D–shape matching is transformed into measuring similarity between 2D–shapes. The shape descriptor is defined by the set of the k largest singular values of the 2D images and Euclidean distance between the vector descriptors is used as a similarity measure. The preliminary results obtained on a simple database show promising performance with a mean average precision (MAP) of 0.82 and could allow using the approach as part of a retrieval system in clinical routine.

Keywords: 2D–based 3D retrieval · Region detector · Singular value decomposition

1 Introduction

Radiologists are dealing with an increasing number and also a strongly increasing variety of medical images [1,2]. Imaging techniques are an essential part of diagnosis and treatment planning. Many physicians also have regular information needs during clinical work, teaching preparation and research activities [3,4], where computerized tools can help make the search more efficient and effective. Medical image retrieval has been an area of intensive research for the past 20 years [2,5] and 3D data access has started to get increasing attention, as it is the medical imaging modality that is increasing fastest in terms of data produced. The need to search for 3D volumes using their visual content to complement textual search in annotations has led to the development of several approaches to compute similarity between two 3D volumes in recent years [6]. Users can search for 3D volumes by supplying an example query volume or mark a volume of interest. Several articles describe these types of image search [7]. In this

B. Menze et al. (Eds.): MCV 2013, LNCS 8331, pp. 185–195, 2014.
DOI: 10.1007/978-3-319-05530-5_18, © Springer International Publishing Switzerland 2014

paper, we propose a novel 3D retrieval model to retrieve medical volumes using 2D images as input. This is intuitive as 2D images might be available easily as a starting point for queries, for example via images in the literature, images used in scientific presentations or for teaching. Medical image databases often contain images of many different modalities, taken under varied conditions [8]. The 2D–based 3D retrieval also provides numerous opportunities for working between 2D modalities such as x–ray and 3D modalities such as CT. However, many current 2D approaches to search for 3D volumes are based on retrieval by sketch [6, 9, 10]. Most applications of 2D–based 3D volume retrieval focus on objects [11, 12] and not on medical images where generally solid texture and not an object surface is the target for search.

When retrieving 3D volumes using 2D query images that are not necessarily single slices of a volume, we need to compute the distance between the query image and the 3D volumes in the database. The algorithm we propose is composed of four stages:

- region detection in 3D volumes;
- volume projection onto 2D planes;
- singular value extraction from the projections;
- similarity calculation between a query and the projections.

Conventionally, regions of interest for retrieval are detected using algorithms such as the Sobel filter, Prewitt algorithm or Laplacian of Gaussian [13]. In the first step of our approach, a region of interest detector for medical images is applied that is able to provide locally salient regions at various scales [7].

The binary 3D images with the regions detected are then associated with three canonical 2D projections at each of the scales. A few 3D retrieval approaches using 2D projection views have also been proposed recently [11, 12]. Most of them use polyhedron–based views [14] for the projections. In the approach presented in this paper canonical projections are used because medical images are usually created using very standardized acquisition settings. As a result we obtain the 2D silhouette views of the volumes. We then have a simpler binary 2D silhouette retrieval problem. To compute the distance between two views, we need to extract an appropriate shape descriptor. Each image is processed in order to extract and describe the shape of the regions. The shape descriptor we chose is defined by the set of the k largest singular values of the 2D regions. In the literature, singular values were used in the past as shape descriptors for face recognition [15–17]. In order to validate the approach we use a simple database consisting of head and thorax volumes. The Euclidean norm between the shape descriptors is used as similarity measure.

The rest of the paper is organized as follows. In Sect. 2 the database and the methods used on our approach are described. The results are presented in Sect. 3. Section 4 concludes the paper and list several future research ideas.

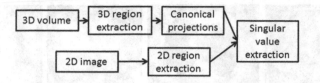

Fig. 1. Schematic overview of the image processing steps of the described approach.

2   Materials and Methods

This section describes the materials and methods used for 2D–based 3D medical image retrieval (see also Fig. 1). Let $I_v \in \mathcal{M}_{m \times n \times o}(\mathbb{R})$ be a volume that is part of the database. The volumes are analyzed as follows:

1. A volume $I_{v_{br}} \in \mathcal{M}_{m \times n \times o}(\{0, 1\})$ with detected binary regions of I_v is created (see Subsect. 2.2 for more details).
2. $I_{v_{br}}$ is projected onto the three canonical axes, P_x, P_y and P_z (see Subsect. 2.3).
3. The k largest singular values of the projections P_x, P_y and P_z are used as shape descriptors (see Subsect. 2.4).

Let $I \in \mathcal{M}_{p \times q}(\mathbb{R})$ be a 2D image that can be used as an example query to find corresponding volumes. The following steps are applied to this image:

1. An image $I_{br} \in \mathcal{M}_{p \times q}(\{0, 1\})$ with detected binary regions I is created (see Subsect. 2.2).
2. The k largest singular values of the image with the detected regions I_{br} are used as shape descriptor (see Subsect. 2.4).

Finally, the distance between the singular values of the 2D and of each of the three projections of the 3D volume are calculated. Only the nearest projection is used for the retrieval step (see Subsect. 2.5). In the following subsections the steps are described in more detail.

2.1   Database

To carry out this preliminary study and show the feasibility of the approach, images from three existing databases are used (two databases to create a set of volumes and one database to get 2D query images). All the volumes of the two databases are images taken for research from clinical routine:

- 41 T1 and T2 weighted head MRI series were used. All images were acquired on a 3T MR imaging scanner (Magnetom Trio a Tim System, Siemens, Germany) using a head coil.
- 41 thorax CTs were used, acquired on a GE DECT (General Electrics Dual Energy Computed Tomography) scanner; only one energy level was used.

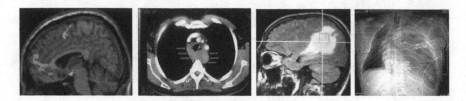

Fig. 2. Sample images used from ImageCLEF data set.

2D images from the same anatomic regions as the selected 3D volumes (head, chest) were chosen from the publicly available ImageCLEF medical database [18] as query images. This database consists of images from articles of the biomedical open access literature from various modalities (CT and MRI slices, x–ray images, etc.). Since the images belong to scientific articles many of them contain annotations such as colored arrows or are cropped and modified in many other ways (see Fig. 2). Images can be of different modalities than the volumes for the same anatomic region and in differing level/window settings. In total, 95 2D query images were used (47 of the head and 48 of the thorax). The 2D database was divided into two subsets, a training set to optimize the parameters (24 of the head and 24 of the thorax) and a test set for showing the stability of the approach (23 of the head and 24 of the thorax). The query images contain also other modalities than the volumes, for example chest x–rays to search for chest CT volumes.

2.2   Region Detection

A key–region detector [7] is applied providing locally relevant regions of interest based on the actual patterns of the image with no predefined shape. The key–region detector is based on a wavelet pyramid, providing meaningful regions at various scales. We can use the same algorithm to detect regions in 3D as well as in 2D (see Fig. 3) due to the dimensionality–independence of the detector. The algorithm automatically detects salient regions at various scales. Two examples

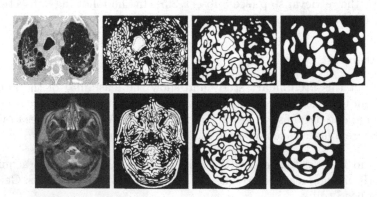

Fig. 3. 2D images and their detected regions at the scales 4, 8 and 16.

showing the regions detected in 2D images are illustrated in Fig. 3. Figure 4(d) shows the regions detected in a volume.

2.3   Projections

The projection step aims at extracting a 2D representation of the binary 3D volumes to be able to compare them with the 2D queries. To compute the view of a 3D volume on a plain, we extract the projections along the three canonical axes (x, y and z) [19]. Canonical projections are used as the acquisition protocol of the medical volumes is fully standardized and usually has these same projections. The projections of a binary region image $I_{v_{br}}(x, y, z) \in \mathcal{M}_{m \times n \times o}(\{0, 1\})$ are (see Fig. 4(a), (b) and (c)):

$$P_x(y_0, z_0) = \begin{cases} 1 \ if \ \exists x/I_{v_{br}}(x, y_0, z_0) = 1 \\ 0 \ \ \text{otherwise} \end{cases} , \text{ for } 0 < y_0 < N, 0 < z_0 < O \quad (1)$$

$$P_y(x_0, z_0) = \begin{cases} 1 \ if \ \exists y/I_{v_{br}}(x_0, y, z_0) = 1 \\ 0 \ \text{otherwise} \end{cases} , \text{ for } 0 < x_0 < M, 0 < z_0 < O \quad (2)$$

$$P_z(x_0, y_0) = \begin{cases} 1 \ if \ \exists z/I_{v_{br}}(x_0, y_0, z) = 1 \\ 0 \ \text{otherwise} \end{cases} , \text{ for } 0 < x_0 < M, 0 < y_0 < N \quad (3)$$

2.4   Singular Value Decomposition

The singular value decomposition (SVD) of a rectangular matrix $A \in \mathcal{M}_{m \times n}(\mathbb{R})$ is decomposed in the form [20]:

$$A = UDV^T \quad (4)$$

where $U \in \mathcal{M}_{m \times m}(\mathbb{R})$ and $V \in \mathcal{M}_{n \times n}(\mathbb{R})$ are orthogonal matrices. The singular values of A, $\sigma_1 \geq \sigma_2, ... \geq \sigma_p \geq 0$ with $p = min\{m, n\}$, appear in descending order along the main diagonal D.

By applying a singular value decomposition, the matrix can be decomposed into a matrix that contains intrinsic shape information, the singular value matrix D, and matrices with information about corresponding points U and V. An important property of the SVD is that the largest singular values in D always hold the maximum possible information and show stability for most image modifications [21] because of its geometrical invariance [21]. We use a set of k largest singular values of the binary images as a shape descriptor. The truncated SVD captures most of the underlying structure and at the same time removes noise [22].

2.5   Comparison

We measure the effectiveness of our approach using 2D images as queries and 3D volumes as the database and anatomic region as the ground truth. To assess the overall performance of our algorithm, we test our retrieval algorithm on the

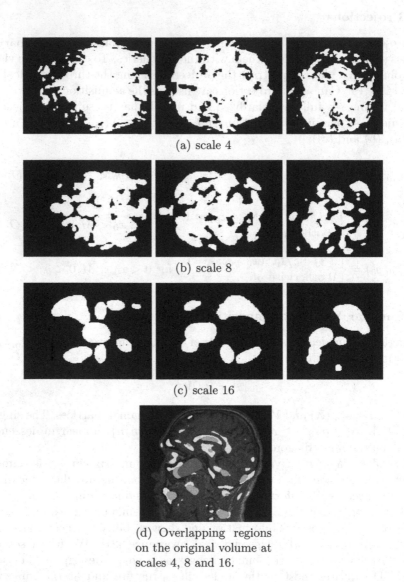

(a) scale 4

(b) scale 8

(c) scale 16

(d) Overlapping regions
on the original volume at
scales 4, 8 and 16.

Fig. 4. 2D binary projections at various scales; original volume with regions detected.

complete training query set. The parameters which achieved the best results over the training data were used for evaluation on the test data. Separation between test and training data set is random, respecting that both contain an equal number of instances from each anatomic region. In order to measure the quality of the retrieval, the average precision (AveP) is calculated for each query to get an overall picture of the quality in such a simple retrieval scenario. Then, the mean value of the average precision scores from all the queries is calculated (MAP) [23]. There are many evaluation methods proposed in image retrieval to evaluate the effectiveness of the systems [24]. MAP was chosen as it is a standard measure in the main information retrieval benchmarks [25]. MAP scores were also measured for various similarity distances over the training set.

3   Results

We implement a 2D–based 3D volume retrieval system based on the proposed framework. The subjects of the 2D views are not the same as the 3D volumes and the task is harder as the views can vary strongly and can be cropped and modified in many ways. The performance of this scenario is measured by the MAP of the volumes retrieved when 2D images are taken as queries. For our experiments over the test set the 10 largest singular values from the scale 4 were used. These parameters were taken from an analysis on the training set. The

Table 1. MAP using various scales and the k largest singular values on the training set using Euclidean distance.

scale \ k	3	5	10	15	25	50
2	0.5264	0.5655	0.6574	0.6775	0.6645	0.6518
4	0.6623	0.7251	**0.7646**	0.7150	0.6462	0.6478
8	0.6153	0.6116	0.59011	0.5814	0.5767	0.5656
16	0.5310	0.5405	0.5503	0.5579	0.5712	0.5875
32	0.5598	0.5696	0.5585	0.5529	0.5578	0.5634
64	0.6893	0.6894	0.6894	0.6894	0.6894	0.6894

Table 2. MAP using various scales and the k largest singular values on the training set using Canberra distance.

scale \ k	3	5	10	15	25	50
2	0.5403	0.5841	0.6606	0.6906	0.7048	0.6514
4	0.6360	0.6547	0.6653	0.6691	0.6652	0.6599
8	0.6179	0.6367	0.6149	0.6248	0.6394	0.6432
16	0.5606	0.5493	0.5399	0.5598	0.5828	0.6137
32	0.5578	0.5519	0.5555	0.5480	0.6151	0.6326
64	**0.7073**	0.6895	0.6621	0.6361	0.5897	0.5897

Table 3. MAP using various scales and the k largest singular values on the training set using chi–square distance.

scale \ k	3	5	10	15	25	50
2	0.5390	0.5831	0.6839	0.6790	0.6490	0.6523
4	0.6422	0.6761	**0.7511**	0.7278	0.6632	0.650
8	0.6126	0.6180	0.6012	0.5972	0.5883	0.5814
16	0.5456	0.5434	0.5536	0.5519	0.5495	0.5707
32	0.5630	0.6126	0.5904	0.5582	0.5674	0.5644
64	0.6881	0.6881	0.6881	0.6881	0.6881	0.6881

Table 4. MAP using various scales and the k largest singular values on the training set using cosine similarity.

scale \ k	3	5	10	15	25	50
2	0.6184	0.5622	0.5620	0.5900	0.6290	0.6486
4	0.6528	0.6528	0.6529	0.6529	0.6531	0.6536
8	0.6203	0.6061	0.5753	0.5652	0.5550	0.5516
16	0.5287	0.5281	0.5309	0.5323	0.5348	0.5549
32	0.5422	0.5396	0.5532	0.5357	0.5563	0.5618
64	**0.6986**	**0.6986**	**0.6986**	**0.6986**	**0.69863**	**0.69863**

Table 5. MAP using various scales and the k largest singular values on the training set using histogram intersection.

scale \ k	3	5	10	15	25	50
2	0.5291	0.5718	0.6659	0.6821	0.6615	0.6527
4	0.6388	0.7146	**0.7512**	0.7249	0.6491	0.6533
8	0.5966	0.6141	0.5964	0.5782	0.5696	0.5618
16	0.5575	0.5633	0.5812	0.5973	0.6096	0.6106
32	0.5512	0.5553	0.5634	0.5738	0.5671	0.5723
64	0.6986	0.69863	0.69863	0.69863	0.69863	0.69863

approach achieves a MAP of **0.8236** on the test data, showing the stability of the approach. In the analysis over the training set we tested various similarity measures: Euclidean distance (Table 1), Canberra distance (Table 2), chi–square distance (Table 3), cosine similarity (Table 4), histogram intersection (Table 5) and Jeffrey divergence (Table 6). The results show that using the Euclidean distance the best results are achieved. For this reason Euclidean distance was used to evaluate MAP over the test data.

Table 6. MAP using various scales and the k largest singular values on the training set using Jeffrey divergence.

scale \ k	3	5	10	15	25	50
2	0.5530	0.5921	0.6934	0.6789	0.6565	0.6565
4	0.6421	0.6786	**0.7519**	0.7260	0.6565	0.6565
8	0.6173	0.6234	0.6029	0.6595	0.6565	0.6565
16	0.5443	0.5406	0.5702	0.6319	0.6565	0.6565
32	0.5758	0.6211	0.6082	0.6553	0.6565	0.6565
64	0.6894	0.6894	0.6894	0.6894	0.6894	0.6894

4   Conclusions and Future Work

This paper describes an approach for 2D–based 3D retrieval in medical databases. Such a system can be useful for clinicians searching for volumes when they have a single 2D view of an image available, for example from a 2D modality, a medical article or from a PowerPoint presentation.

The preliminary results obtained show promising performance with a MAP of 0.82 and allow using the approach as part of a retrieval system for clinical routine. This shows that most images of the same anatomic region can be identified even when queries are not of the same modality or are cropped and otherwise modified. Using 2D images as queries to retrieve 3D volumes may provide a useful tool for radiologists searching for information on specific regions of interest. Obviously, the current scenario of using only two anatomic regions is a very simplified scenario. It is planned to extend the approach to a much larger set of anatomic regions. Larger databases are currently being created and should be directly usable with the same approach. In terms of relevance for specific information needs it is also clear that not only anatomy are important but also local characteristics representing pathologies. Still the described approach already allows filtering out similar anatomic regions that can then be further exploited for visually similar regions of interest. The approach is a step towards retrieval between images of differing dimensionality.

Acknowledgments. The research leading to these results has received funding from the European Union's Seventh Framework Programme under grant agreement 257528 (KHRESMOI) and 258191 (PROMISE). The authors would like to thanks also the project TEC2012-39095-C03-02, of the Spanish Ministry of Economy and Competitiveness.

References

1. Akgül, C., Rubin, D., Napel, S., Beaulieu, C., Greenspan, H., Acar, B.: Content-based image retrieval in radiology: current status and future directions. J. Digit. Imaging **24**(2), 208–222 (2011)

2. Hwang, K.H., Lee, H., Choi, D.: Medical image retrieval: past and present. Health Inf. Res. **18**(1), 3–9 (2012)

3. Hersh, W., Jensen, J., Müller, H., Gorman, P., Ruch, P.: A qualitative task analysis for developing an image retrieval test collection. In: ImageCLEF/MUSCLE Workshop on Image Retrieval Evaluation, Vienna, Austria, pp. 11–16 (2005)

4. Müller, H., Despont-Gros, C., Hersh, W., Jensen, J., Lovis, C., Geissbuhler, A.: Health care professionals' image use and search behaviour. In: Proceedings of the Medical Informatics Europe Conference (MIE 2006), pp. 24–32. IOS Press, Studies in Health Technology and Informatics, Maastricht, The Netherlands, August 2006

5. Müller, H., Michoux, N., Bandon, D., Geissbuhler, A.: A review of content-based image retrieval systems in medicine-clinical benefits and future directions. Int. J. Med. Inform. **73**(1), 1–23 (2004)

6. Yoon, S.M., Scherer, M., Schreck, T., Kuijper, A.: Sketch-based 3D model retrieval using diffusion tensor fields of suggestive contours. In: ACM Multimedia, pp. 193–200 (2010)

7. Foncubierta-Rodríguez, A., Müller, H., Depeursinge, A.: Region-based volumetric medical image retrieval. In: Law, M.Y., Boonn, W.W. (eds.) SPIE Medical Imaging: Advanced PACS-Based Imaging Informatics and Therapeutic Applications. SPIE, Belgium (2013)

8. Kalpathy-Cramer, J., Hersh, W.: Medical image retrieval and automatic annotation: OHSU at ImageCLEF 2007. In: Peters, C., Jijkoun, V., Mandl, T., Müller, H., Oard, D.W., Peñas, A., Petras, V., Santos, D. (eds.) CLEF 2007. LNCS, vol. 5152, pp. 623–630. Springer, Heidelberg (2008)

9. Pu, J., Ramani, K.: A 3D model retrieval method using 2D freehand sketches. In: Sunderam, V.S., van Albada, G.D., Sloot, P.M.A., Dongarra, J.J. (eds.) ICCS 2005. LNCS, vol. 3515, pp. 343–346. Springer, Heidelberg (2005)

10. Li, B., Johan, H.: Sketch-based 3D model retrieval by incorporating 2D–3D alignment. Multimedia Tools Appl. **65**(3), 363–385 (2013)

11. Napoléon, T., Sahbi, H.: Content-based 3D object retrieval using 2D views. In: Proceedings of the International Conference on Image Processing, ICIP'09, pp. 1437–1440 (2009)

12. Petre, R.D., Zaharia, T., Prêteux, F.: An overview of view-based 2D/3D indexing methods. In: SPIE Mathematics of Data/Image Coding, Compression, and Encryption with Applications XII, vol. 7799 (2010)

13. Yu-qian, Z., Wei-hua, G., Zhen-cheng, C., Jing-tian, T., Ling-yun, L.: Medical images edge detection based on mathematical morphology. In: Proceedings of the 2005 IEEE Engineering in Medicine and Biology 27th Annual Conference (2005)

14. Xiao, H., Zhang, X.: A method for content-based 3D model retrieval by 2D projection views. WSEAS Trans. Circuits Syst. **7**(5), 445–449 (2008)

15. Smeets, D., Fabry, T., Hermans, J., Vandermeulen, D., Suetens, P.: Isometric deformation modeling using singular value decomposition for 3D expression-invariant face recognition. In: IEEE 3rd International Conference on Biometrics: Theory, Applications and Systems, BTAS '09, pp. 1–6 (2009)

16. Smeets, D., Hermans, J., Vandermeulen, D., Suetens, P.: Isometric deformation invariant 3D shape recognition. Pattern Recogn. **45**(7), 2817–2831 (2012)

17. Wang, Y., Wang, Y., Jain, A.K., Tan, T.: Face verification based on bagging RBF networks. In: Zhang, D., Jain, A.K. (eds.) ICB 2005. LNCS, vol. 3832, pp. 69–77. Springer, Heidelberg (2005)

18. Müller, H., García Seco de Herrera, A., Kalpathy-Cramer, J., Demner Fushman, D., Antani, S., Eggel, I.: Overview of the imageCLEF 2012 medical image retrieval and classification tasks. In: Working Notes of CLEF 2012 (Cross Language, Evaluation Forum), September 2012
19. Lehmann, G.: Image projections along an axis. Insight J. (2006)
20. Golub, G.H., van Loan, C.F.: Matrix Computations (1996)
21. Jiao, Y., Yang, B., Wang, H., Niu, X.: SVD based robust image content retrieval. In: Proceedings of the 2006 International Conference on Intelligent Information Hiding and Multimedia, IIH-MSP '06, pp. 351–354 (2006)
22. Berry, M.W., Dumais, S.T., O'Brien, G.W.: Using linear algebra for intelligent information retrieval. SIAM Rev. **37**(4), 573–595 (1995)
23. Kishida, K.: Property of average precision and its generalization: an examination of evaluation indicator for information retrieval experiments. Technical report, National Institute of Informatics, Tokyo, Japan (2005)
24. Volk, M., Ripplinger, B., Vintar, S., Buitelaar, P., Raileanu, D., Sacaleanu, B.: Semantic annotation for concept-based cross-language medical information retrieval. Int. J. Med. Inform. **67**, 97–112 (2002)
25. Voorhees, E.M., Harman, D.K.: TREC: Experiment and Evaluation in Information Retrieval. MIT press, Cambridge (2005)

Feature Extraction with Intrinsic Distortion Correction in Celiac Disease Imagery: No Need for Rasterization

Michael Gadermayr[1](✉), Andreas Uhl[1], and Andreas Vécsei[2]

[1] Department of Computer Sciences, University of Salzburg, Salzburg, Austria
{mgadermayr,uhl}@cosy.sbg.ac.at
http://www.wavelab.at
[2] Endoscopy Unit, St. Anna Children's Hospital, Vienna, Austria

Abstract. In the fields of computer aided celiac disease diagnosis, wide-angle endoscopy lenses are employed which introduce a significant degree of barrel type distortion. In recent studies on celiac disease classification, distortion correction techniques are investigated which use interpolation techniques, in order to maintain the rasterization of the image. Subsequent feature extraction is based on the new images. We introduce a generic feature extraction methodology with intrinsic distortion correction, which does not include this rasterization for features which do not need a regular grid. As distortion correction turned out to be disadvantageous in most cases, we aim in investigating the (negative) effect of the applied rasterization. In our experiments, the omission of rasterization actually turns out to be advantageous. This fact is an incentive for developing more features, which are not based on a regular grid.

1 Introduction

Celiac disease is an autoimmune disorder that affects the small bowel in genetically predisposed individuals of all age groups after introduction of gluten containing food. Characteristic for this disease is an inflammatory reaction in the mucosa of the small intestine caused by a dysregulated immune response triggered by ingested gluten proteins of certain cereals, especially against gliadine. During the course of the disease the mucosa looses its absorptive villi and hyperplasia of the enteric crypts occurs leading to a diminished ability to absorb nutrients. Computer aided celiac disease diagnosis relies on images taken during endoscopy. The employed cameras are equipped with wide angle lenses, which suffer from a significant amount of barrel type distortion. Whereas the distortion in central image pixels can be neglected, peripheral regions are highly distorted. Thereby, the feature extraction as well as the following classification is compromised. Based on camera calibration, distortion correction (DC) techniques are able to rectify the images.

In recent studies, the impact of barrel type distortion [1] and distortion correction [2] on the classification rate of celiac disease endoscopy images has been

B. Menze et al. (Eds.): MCV 2013, LNCS 8331, pp. 196–204, 2014.
DOI: 10.1007/978-3-319-05530-5_19, © Springer International Publishing Switzerland 2014

investigated. The authors showed that image patches in peripheral regions, which are stronger affected by the distortion are more likely to be misclassified. However, with distortion correction, the classification rate on average even suffers. In [3] and [4], different distortion correction techniques and in [5] additionally various interpolation methods have been investigated.

Applying traditional distortion correction introduces the following advantages (+) and disadvantages (−):

- **Geometrical correctness (+):**
  The geometrical relations are rectified.
- **Interpolation within rasterization (−):**
  As the mapping from distorted to undistorted points usually does not result in discrete points, interpolation is necessary.
- **Lack of data points in peripheral regions (−):**
  Due to the stretching of the image points, in peripheral regions, less real data points are available.

In this work, we introduce a generic method to extract distortion corrected features without the need of a previous rasterization. In order to measure the (negative) effect of interpolation in rasterization, the new approach is compared with the traditional feature extraction based on distortion corrected images. Moreover, we compare the new approach with the method based on distorted images which turned out to be mostly advantageous in recent work [2]. In experiments, the competitiveness of the new approach is confirmed. We have to point out, that the proposed approach requires features which are not based on a regular grid, as otherwise the advantage would vanish. In experiments, we show that the proposed intrinsic approach definitely is advantageous compared to the traditional approach based on DC images and for certain setups it is advantageous compared to the approach based on original images.

The paper is organized as follows: In Sect. 2, the traditional way of distortion corrected feature extraction and the new intrinsic technique is explained. In Sect. 3, experiments are shown and the results are discussed. Section 4 concludes this paper.

2   Theory

2.1   Distortion Model

We utilize the distortion correction approach based on the work of Melo et al. [6]. In this approach, the circular barrel type distortion is modeled by the division model [7]. Having the center of distortion $\hat{x}_c$ and the distortion parameter ξ, undistortion (DC) of distorted points x_d and distortion (D) of undistorted points x_u is calculated as follows:

$$DC(x_d) = \hat{x}_c + \frac{(x_d - \hat{x}_c)}{||x_d - \hat{x}_c||_2} \cdot r_u(||x_d - \hat{x}_c||_2) \ . \tag{1}$$

$$D(x_u) = \hat{x}_c + \frac{(x_u - \hat{x}_c)}{||x_u - \hat{x}_c||_2} \cdot r_u^{-1}(||x_u - \hat{x}_c||_2) \,. \tag{2}$$

$||x - \hat{x}_c||_2$ (in the following r) is the distance (radius) of the point x from the center of distortion $\hat{x}_c$. The function r_u defines for a radius r in the distorted image, the new radius in the undistorted image (for distortion (D), the inverse function r_u^{-1} is required):

$$r_u(r) = \frac{r}{1 + \xi \cdot r^2} \,. \tag{3}$$

This approach is very robust, as only the parameters $\hat{x}_c$ and ξ have to be estimated.

2.2   Traditional Distortion Correction in Feature Extraction

In recent studies [1–3], first the undistorted image I_u is computed from the distorted image I_d. Intuitively, for each point x_u in the undistorted image, the corresponding point x_d in the distorted image must be known. However, as $I_d(x_d)$ exists only for discrete points, the simple assumption $I_u(x_u) = I_d(D(x_u))$ does not hold in general (as $D(x_u)$ not necessarily is a discrete point).

First, a continuous signal $I_{d_{cont}}$ must be generated from I_d by e.g. a linear interpolation method:

$$I_{d_{cont}}(x) = \sum_{z \in N} I_d(z) \cdot K(x - z) \,. \tag{4}$$

N is a set of discrete neighbors of x and K is an arbitrary interpolation kernel. Having the continuous signal, the undistorted image can be computed as follows:

$$I_u(x_u) = I_{d_{cont}}(D(x_u)) \,. \tag{5}$$

The distortion corrected feature extraction is executed in the traditional way, based on the undistorted image I_u.

2.3   Intrinsic Distortion Correction

In the tradition approach, before the feature extraction is applied, the undistorted image is generated. Thereby, the feature extraction can be executed in the usual way, as in the new image the rasterization is retrieved. We introduce a feature extraction methodology with intrinsic DC, which is not based on a re-rasterization.

The main idea of intrinsic distortion correction is explained in the following. We introduce two operations, which preserve geometrical correctness, although pixel values are extracted from the distorted image.

Let x_d be a reference point in the distorted image and v be an arbitrary offset vector. $x_d \oplus v$ adds a vector to a point in the image in consideration of geometrical correctness. Both, the original and the resulting point are coordinates of the distorted image:

$$x_d \oplus v = D(DC(x_d) + v) \, . \tag{6}$$

Otherwise, if two distorted reference points x_{d_1} and x_{d_2} are given, the geometrically correct offset vector can be computed as follows:

$$x_{d_1} \ominus x_{d_2} = DC(x_{d_1}) - DC(x_{d_2}) \, . \tag{7}$$

Using these two operations, each feature can be extracted, theoretically. However, although even a regular grid could be created by adding discrete offset vector $(v = (0,1),(1,1),(1,0),(0,2)...)$ to a reference point, intrinsic feature extraction is only sensible if a regular grid is not required. If a grid was essential, interpolation would be necessary in the same way as with the traditional DC.

Features. Many features are based on regular grids (e.g. Fourier based and wavelet based features). We identified the following features, being not based on regular grids:

- Local binary patterns [8] (**LBP**)
- Local ternary patterns [9] (**LTP**)
- Rotational invariant Local binary patterns [10] (**RLBP**)

For computing these features, each (reference) point is encircled by a given number of equidistant circularly arranged samples with a defined radius. The

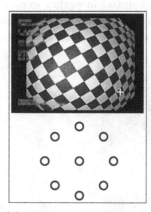 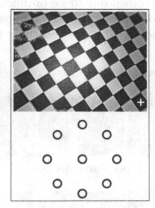 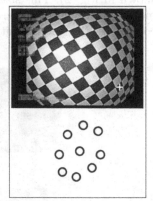

(a) Without DC: Feature extraction based on distorted images with a regular LBP operator.

(b) Traditional DC: Feature extraction based on undistorted images with a regular LBP (Sect. 2.2).

(c) Intrinsic DC: Feature extraction based on distorted images, with a distorted LBP operator (Sect. 2.3).

Fig. 1. The three different feature extraction methodologies are illustrated with a checkerboard image. The top column shows the utilized images and the bottom column shows the applied enlarged LBP templates at the marked point (+).

important thing is, that the exact positions of the samples do not necessarily comply with a regular image raster. That means, in each case, interpolation in feature extraction is required. If the traditional DC approach is utilized, interpolation is applied twice (in rasterization and in feature extraction). With our intrinsic approach, one interpolation step can be avoided. We exploit the operation $\oplus$, to get the neighboring points for each center patch, by adding vectors v with a specific length (which is the radius of LBP) and different directions (directly from the original image).

In Fig. 1, the approaches based on the distorted (Fig. 1a) and undistorted images (Fig. 1b) and the intrinsic approach (Fig. 1c) are illustrated.

Whereas most texture features are based on regular grids new features could be developed which directly exploit the operations $\oplus$ and $\ominus$. Moreover, existing features which are based on regular grids can be modified.

3   Experiments

3.1   Experimental Setup

The image test set used contains images of the Duodenal Bulb taken during duodenoscopies at the St. Anna Children's Hospital using pediatric gastroscopes (with resolution 768×576 and 528×522 pixels, respectively). The mean age of the patients undergoing endoscopy was 11.1 years (range 0.8–20.9 years). The female to male ratio was 1.43:1. In a preprocessing step, texture patches with a fixed size of 128×128 pixels were extracted in a manual fashion (examples are shown in Fig. 2). This size turned out to be optimally suited in earlier experiments on automated celiac disease diagnosis [11]. In case of traditional distortion correction, the patch position is adjusted according to the distortion function.

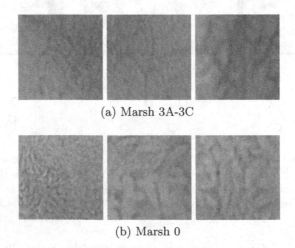

(a) Marsh 3A-3C

(b) Marsh 0

Fig. 2. Example patches of patients with (a) and without the disease (b). In Fig. 2a, the villous structure (b) is missing and only blood vessels can be seen.

With the intrinsic distortion correction, the original patches are preserved. In traditional distortion correction, as well as in feature extraction, bi-linear interpolation is utilized. In our experiments, for feature extraction the patches are converted to gray value images.

To generate the ground truth for the texture patches used, the condition of the mucosal areas covered by the images was determined by histological examination of biopsies from the corresponding regions. Severity of villous atrophy was classified according to the modified Marsh classification in [12].

Although it is possible to distinguish between the different stages of the disease (called Marsh 3A-3C), we only aim in distinguishing between images of patients with (Marsh 3A-3C) and without the disease (called Marsh0). Our experiments are based on a database containing 163 (Marsh 0) and 124 (Marsh 3A-3C) images, respectively. As we do not have a separate evaluation set, leave-one-patient-out cross validation is utilized. Thereby we also do not apply any feature subset selection, but instead evaluate various setups with the features mentioned above. For classification, the k-nearest neighbor classifier is used. We utilize this rather simple classifier in order to focus on the feature extraction stage.

3.2   Results

In Fig. 3a–c, the results of our Experiments are shown. In each plot for one feature and each configuration (applied on the x-axis), 2 bars are shown. A configuration consists of the radius (first value which is reaching from 1 to 4 pixels) and the number of samples (second value which is reaching from 4 to 10). The bold vertical lines separate the considered radii. Whereas the dark-colored left bars indicate the differences of the classification rates between the intrinsic DC approach and the traditional DC approach, the light-colored right bars indicate the differences between the intrinsic DC and the original approach without distortion correction. A positive value means that the classification rate of the new intrinsic method is higher compared to the other method. The value on top of each column shows the classification rate achieved with the original approach without DC. Adding the respective difference, the absolute classification rates of the intrinsic DC method can be estimated. It can be seen, that the left (dark-colored) bars are almost always above zero. That means, the classification rate definitely benefits from our new intrinsic DC approach compared to the traditional DC approach. The behavior of the right (light-colored) bars seems to depend on the considered neighborhood (i.e. the radius). If radius 1 is chosen, intrinsic DC is disadvantageous compared to the approach without DC for each feature and each number of samples. However, in case of larger neighborhoods (especially if radius is 3 or 4), the intrinsic DC turns out to be the better choice as far as the classification rate is concerned. The overall best achieved classification rates for each feature and each DC method are shown in Table 1.

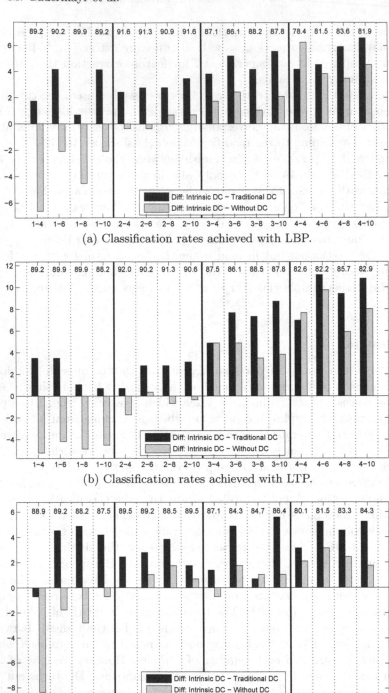

(a) Classification rates achieved with LBP.

(b) Classification rates achieved with LTP.

(c) Classification rates achieved with RLBP.

Fig. 3. Classification rates achieved with the different features.

Table 1. Best configurations for each feature and each DC method.

Feature	DC method	Radius	Samples	Rate
	Without DC	2	8	91.64
LBP	Traditional DC	2	10	88.85
	Intrinsic DC	2	10	**92.33**
	Without DC	2	4	91.99
LTP	Traditional DC	2	4	89.55
	Intrinsic DC	3	4	**92.33**
	Without DC	2	4	89.55
RLBP	Traditional DC	2	6	87.46
	Intrinsic DC	2	8	**90.24**

3.3 Discussion

The new intrinsic DC method definitely is superior to the traditional DC app-roach. The omitted additional interpolation within rasterization improves the classification rate in nearly each case, especially if larger radii are considered. In comparison with the approach based on the original image, the intrinsic DC approach profits from larger radii. If larger radii are considered, the geometrical correctness takes precedence over the lack of data points. In opposite if small radii are considered, the geometrical (in)correctness has less impact than the missing data points. For an extended discussion on the impact of lens distortion correction on feature extraction and following classification we refer to [5]. With 3 out of the 3 tested features, the best overall classification rates are achieved with the intrinsic DC method.

4 Conclusion

With the introduced distortion correction intrinsic feature extraction, the rasterization which is applied in traditional distortion correction can be omitted for specific features. We show, that the classification rate of celiac disease images benefits from the better preservation of information. A benefit is achieved on the one hand if compared to the traditional DC approach. On the other hand, compared with the approach based on original images, intrin-sic DC is advantageous especially if larger neighborhoods are considered. This is an incentive for developing more features which are not based on a regular raster.

Acknowledgment. This work is partially funded by the Austrian Science Fund (FWF) under (Project No. 24366).

References

1. Liedlgruber, M., Uhl, A., Vécsei, A.: Statistical analysis of the impact of distortion (correction) on an automated classification of celiac disease. In: Proceedings of the 17th International Conference on Digital Signal Processing (DSP'11), Corfu, Greece (2011)
2. Gschwandtner, M., Liedlgruber, M., Uhl, A., Vécsei, A.: Experimental study on the impact of endoscope distortion correction on computer-assisted celiac disease diagnosis. In: Proceedings of the 10th International Conference on Information Technology and Applications in Biomedicine (ITAB'10), Corfu, Greece (2010)
3. Gschwandtner, M., Hämmerle-Uhl, J., Höller, Y., Liedlgruber, M., Uhl, A., Vécsei, A.: Improved endoscope distortion correction does not necessarily enhance mucosa-classification based medical decision support systems. In: Proceedings of the IEEE International Workshop on Multimedia, Signal Processing (MMSP'12), pp. 158–163 (2012)
4. Hämmerle-Uhl, J., Höller, Y., Uhl, A., Vécsei, A.: Endoscope distortion correction does not (easily) improve mucosa-based classification of celiac disease. In: Ayache, N., Delingette, H., Golland, P., Mori, K. (eds.) MICCAI 2012, Part III. LNCS, vol. 7512, pp. 574–581. Springer, Heidelberg (2012)
5. Gadermayr, M., Liedlgruber, M., Uhl, A., Vécsei, A.: Evaluation of different distortion correction methods and interpolation techniques for an automated classification of celiac disease. Comput. Methods Programs Biomed. (2013) accepted
6. Melo, R., Barreto, J.P., Falcao, G.: A new solution for camera calibration and real-time image distortion correction in medical endoscopy-initial technical evaluation. IEEE Trans. Biomed. Eng. **59**(3), 634–644 (2012)
7. Fitzgibbon, A.W.: Simultaneous linear estimation of multiple view geometry and lens distortion. In: CVPR, pp. 125–132 (2001)
8. Ojala, T., Pietikäinen, M., Harwood, D.: A comparative study of texture measures with classification based on feature distributions. Pattern Recogn. **29**(1), 51–59 (1996)
9. Tan, X., Triggs, B.: Enhanced local texture feature sets for face recognition under difficult lighting conditions. Anal. Model. Faces Gestures **4778**, 168–182 (2007)
10. Ojala, T., Pietikäinen, M., Mäenpää, T.: Multiresolution Gray-Scale and rotation invariant texture classification with local binary patterns. IEEE Trans. Pattern Anal. Mach. Intell. **24**(7), 971–987 (2002)
11. Hegenbart, S., Kwitt, R., Liedlgruber, M., Uhl, A., Vécsei, A.: Impact of duodenal image capturing techniques and duodenal regions on the performance of automated diagnosis of celiac disease. In: Proceedings of the 6th International Symposium on Image and Signal Processing and Analysis (ISPA '09), Salzburg, Austria, pp. 718–723 (2009)
12. Oberhuber, G., Granditsch, G., Vogelsang, H.: The histopathology of coeliac disease: time for a standardized report scheme for pathologists. Eur. J. Gastroenterol. Hepatol. **11**, 1185–1194 (1999)

A Novel Shape Feature Descriptor for the Classification of Polyps in HD Colonoscopy

Michael Häfner[1], Andreas Uhl[2]($\boxtimes$), and Georg Wimmer[2]($\boxtimes$)

[1] St. Elisabeth Hospital, Vienna, Austria
[2] Department of Computer Sciences, University of Salzburg, Salzburg, Austria
{gwimmer,uhl}@cosy.sbg.ac.at

Abstract. This work proposes a new method analyzing the shape of connected components (blobs) from segmented images for the classification of colonic polyps. The segmentation algorithm is a novel variation of the fast level lines transform and the resultant blobs are ideal to model the pit pattern structure of the mucosa. The shape of the blobs is described by a mixture of new features (convex hull, skeletonization and perimeter) as well as already proven features (contrast feature). We show that shape features of blobs extracted by segmenting an image are particularly suitable for mucosal texture classification and outperforming commonly used feature extraction methods.

Additionally this work compares and analyzes the influences of image enhancement technologies to the automated classification of the colonic mucosa. In particular, we compare the conventional chromoendoscopy with the computed virtual chromoendoscopy (the i-Scan technology of Pentax). Results imply that computed virtual chromoendoscopy facilitates the discrimination between healthy and abnormal mucosa, whereas conventional chromoendoscopy rather complicates the discrimination.

Keywords: Computed virtual chromoendoscopy · Chromoendoscopy · i-Scan · Texture recognition · HD-endoscopy · Segmentation · Blob

1 Introduction

Colonic polyps have a rather high prevalence and are known to either develop into cancer or to be precursors of colon cancer. Hence, an early assessment of the malignant potential of such polyps is important as this can lower the mortality rate drastically. As a consequence, a regular colon examination is recommended, especially for people at an age of 50 years and older. The current gold standard for the examination of the colon is colonoscopy, performed by using a colonoscope. Modern endoscopy devices are able to take pictures or videos from inside the colon, allowing to obtain images (or videos) for a computer-assisted analysis with the goal of detecting and diagnosing abnormalities. To enable an easier detection and diagnosis of the extent of a lesion, there are two common image enhancement technologies:

B. Menze et al. (Eds.): MCV 2013, LNCS 8331, pp. 205–213, 2014.
DOI: 10.1007/978-3-319-05530-5_20, © Springer International Publishing Switzerland 2014

1. Conventional chromoendoscopy (CC) came into clinical use 40 years ago. By staining the mucosa using (indigocarmine) dye spray, it is easier to find and classify polyps.
2. Digital chromoendoscopy is a technique to facilitate "chromoendoscopy without dyes" [1]. The strategies followed by major manufacturers differ in this area:
   - In Narrow band imaging (NBI, Olympus), narrow bandpass filters are placed in front of a conventional white-light source to enhance the detail of certain aspects of the surface of the mucosa.
   - The i-Scan (Pentax) image processing technology [2] is a digital contrast method which consists of combinations of surface enhancement (SE), contrast enhancement (CE) and tone enhancement (TE).
   The FICE system (Fujinon) decomposes images by wavelength and then directly reconstructs images with enhanced mucosal surface contrast.
   Both systems (i-Scan and FICE) apply post-processing to the reflected light and thus are called "computed virtual chromoendoscopy (CVC)".

Previous works for the computer assisted staging of colon polyps, which are using endoscopes producing highly detailed images in combination with image enhancement technologies, can be divided in two categories: high-magnification chromoendoscopy ([3]) and high-magnification endoscopy combined with NBI ([4]). In this work we use highly detailed images acquired by a high definition (HD) endoscope without magnification in combination with CC and CVC (the i-Scan technology). To the best of our knowledge, this is the first work for computer assisted colonic polyp classification using HD-endoscopy combined with CVC as well as HD-endoscopy combined with CC. We use three different i-Scan modes:

- i-Scan 1 includes SE and CE. This mode enhances surface and pit pattern details, helping to detect dysplastic areas and to accentuate mucosal surfaces.
- i-Scan 2 includes SE, CE and TE. This mode visually enhances boundaries, margins, surface architecture and hard-to-discern polyps.
- i-Scan 3 also includes SE, CE and TE. This mode is similar to i-Scan 2, with increased illumination and emphasis on the visualization of vascular features.

In Fig. 1 we see an image showing an adenomatous polyp without image enhancement technology (a), example images using CVC (b,c,d), an image using CC (e) and images combining CC and CVC by using the i-Scan technology to visually enhance the already stained mocusa (f,g,h).

In this work we will compare classification results with respect to using CVC (i-Scan) or CC. We will also examine the effects of combinations of CVC and CC on the classification results.

For the classification of the images, we propose a new method analyzing the shape of connected components of segmented images.

To find out which image enhancement technologies are most suitable for the computer-aided mucosal texture classification and to compare the results of our proposed method with methods already proven to be successful, we additionally

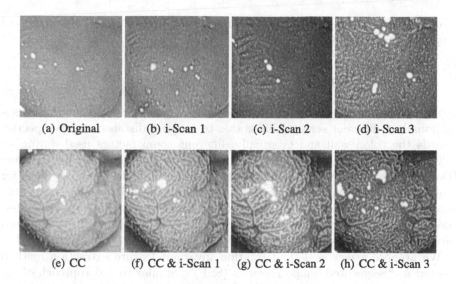

(a) Original   (b) i-Scan 1   (c) i-Scan 2   (d) i-Scan 3

(e) CC   (f) CC & i-Scan 1   (g) CC & i-Scan 2   (h) CC & i-Scan 3

Fig. 1. Images using digital (i-Scan) and/or conventional chromoendoscopy (CC)

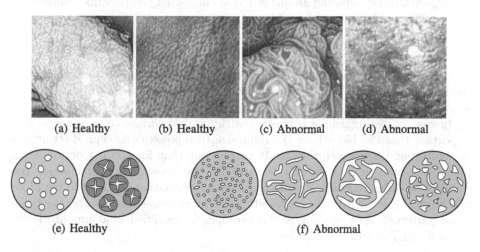

(a) Healthy   (b) Healthy   (c) Abnormal   (d) Abnormal

(e) Healthy   (f) Abnormal

Fig. 2. Example images of the two classes (a–d) and the pit pattern types of these two classes (e–f)

employ a number of well known feature extraction methods for the classification of mucosal texture.

We differentiate between two classes, normal mucosa or hyperplastic polyps (class healthy) and neoplastic, adenomatous or carcinomatous structures (class abnormal) (see Fig. 2a–d). The various pit pattern types [5] of these two classes are presented in Fig. 2e–f.

This paper is organized as follows. Section 2 describes the feature extraction methods, especially our new method based on shapes of connected components (blobs). In Sect. 3 we describe the experiments and present the results. Section 4 presents the conclusion.

2   Feature Extraction

In colonoscopic (and other types of endoscopic) imagery, mucosa texture is usually found at different scales. This is due to varying distance and perspective towards the colon wall and eventually different zoom factors used during an endoscopy session. The differences in scale are for example much higher using HD-endoscopes (especially because of the highly variable distance) than for using high-magnification endoscopes, where the distance of the endoscope to the mucosa is relatively constant. Consequently, in order to design reliable computer-aided mucosa texture classification schemes, the scale invariance of the employed feature sets could be essential.

We propose a new scale and rotation invariant feature extraction method denoted as "Segmented Shape Features (SSF)". Similar to the approach of [6], our approach is based on the fast level lines transform (FLLT) [7], which is a fast algorithm decomposing an image I into connected components (blobs S) of upper (X_λ) and lower level set (X^μ):

$$X_\lambda = \{x \in \mathbb{R}^2, I(x) \geq \lambda\}, \qquad X^\mu = \{x \in \mathbb{R}^2, I(x) \leq \mu\}. \qquad (1)$$

By grouping the blobs depending on their size, a scale-space representation is created. The family of blobs S is ordered in a tree structure, showing which blob is contained within another.

In case of distinguishing between healthy and abnormal colon mucosa, it is important that the blobs have the right size to represent the typical structures of healthy and abnormal mucosa. It turned out that for too big or too small blobs it is hard to find suitable features for the classification of images. Too small blobs do not contain any discriminative information and for too big blobs it is hard to extract features representing the local mucosal structure (the types of pit patterns). As a solution of this problem we modified (and simplified) the original FLLT algorithm as follows:

Generating dark (bright) blobs R by localized region growing:

1. Scan the image for a not tagged local minimum (maximum for bright blobs) x_0 with gray value g and create a blob R consisting of only x_0 at the first iteration.
2. Find all neighbors N (4-connectivity) of R with $g_N = \min_{x \in N} I(x)$ ($g_N = \max_{x \in N} I(x)$ for bright blobs) and tag them.
3. Two cases are possible:
    - $g \leq g_N$ ($g \geq g_N$ for bright blobs):
        - $R \leftarrow R \cup \{x \in N | I(x) = g_N\}$
        - $g \leftarrow g_N$
        - Return to step 2.

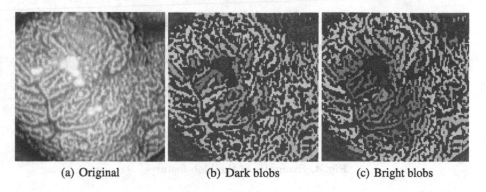

(a) Original   (b) Dark blobs   (c) Bright blobs

Fig. 3. The extracted dark and bright blobs of the original image (Color figure online)

- $g > g_N$ ($g < g_N$ for bright blobs): Set the gray-levels of the pixels in R to g and go to step 1.

The difference of our simplified FLLT algorithm to that of [7] is that we only record the blobs R when reaching the break condition at step 3 (when $g < g_N$), whereas the original FLLT approach additionally records the R's in step 3 whenever $g < g_N$ (dark blobs) or $g > g_N$ (bright blobs). The original FLLT approach also merges the blobs to bigger blobs resulting in a tree structure of blobs R (with a huge amount of blobs of all possible sizes). For our field of application, it turned out that the blobs R recorded reaching the break condition at the end of step 3 are ideal to distinguish between healthy and abnormal colon mucosa. These dark and bright blobs are well suited (size and shape of the blobs) to model the local pit pattern structure of the mucosa (except for too small blobs –less than 9 pixels– which are not considered for further feature extraction) enabling the distinction between healthy and affected mucosa. In Fig. 3 we see an example image and the corresponding dark and bright blobs located with our simplified algorithm. The color of a blob in Fig. 3 denotes the averaged brightness of the pixels inside the blob (red is bright, blue is dark).

To extract information about the contrast inside of the blobs we compute the contrast feature CF (used in [6]) as follows: For each pixel x contained in a blob R, a normalized gray value is computed as

$$CF(x) = \frac{I(x) - \text{mean}_{R(x)}(I)}{\sqrt{\text{var}_{R(x)}(I)}}, \tag{2}$$

where $R(x)$ is the blob containing x, $\text{mean}_{R(x)}(I)$ and $\text{var}_{R(x)}(I)$ are the mean and the variance of the image I over R, respectively.

The CF is computed separately for pixels contained in dark and bright blobs, respectively. This results in two contrast feature histograms (CFH), computed by scanning all pixels contained in dark or bright blobs.

Additionally we use three new scale and rotation invariant shape features suitable for mucosal texture classification. The convex hull feature (CH) (see

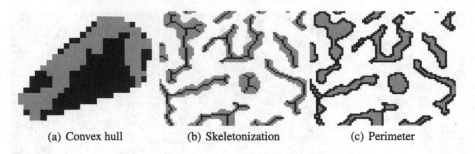

(a) Convex hull   (b) Skeletonization   (c) Perimeter

Fig. 4. Examples of the blob features

Fig. 4) is showing the proportion of the dilation of a blob R to the density of the blob (the number of pixels of R):

$$CH(R) = \frac{\text{\# Pixels of Convex Hull}(R)}{\text{\# Pixels of } R} \tag{3}$$

An example of the convex hull of a blob is shown in Fig. 4. The blob R is shown in gray, the convex hull of R is shown in black and gray.

The skeletonization (SK) and the perimeter (PE) feature (see Fig. 4) are both indicating the flatness of a blob R:

$$SK(R) = \frac{\text{\# Pixels of Skeletonization}(R)}{\sqrt{\text{\# Pixels of } R}}, \quad PE(R) = \frac{\text{\# Pixels of Perimeter}(R)}{\sqrt{\text{\# Pixels of } R}} \tag{4}$$

In Fig. 4, the skeletonizations and the perimeters of the blobs are shown in black and the blobs are shown in gray. The scale invariance of the three shape features is gained by normalizing the shape features (the denominators in Eqs. 3 and 4).

The three shape features are computed separately for dark and bright blobs resulting in 6 shape histograms. The final feature vector of an image consists of the aggregation of the two contrast histograms (25 bins per histogram) and the 6 shape histograms (15 bins per histogram). Each of the four features is able to achieve good results classifying polyps, but the best results are achieved by aggregating the histograms of the four features.

Distances between two feature vectors are measured using the χ^2 statistic which has been frequently used to compare probability distributions (histograms) and is defined by

$$\chi^2(x, y) = \sum_i \frac{(x_i - y_i)^2}{x_i + y_i} \tag{5}$$

Additionally, we employ a number of well known feature extraction methods to compare their results with our SSF method and also to have a higher number of methods resulting in more reliable conclusions with respect to the suitability of the CVC and CC for the automated mucosal texture classification:

DT-CWT [3] is a multi-scale and multi-orientation wavelet transform. The final feature vector of an image consists of the statistical features mean and standard deviation of the absolute values of the subband coefficients (6 decomposition levels × 6 orientations × 3 color channels × 2 features per subband = 216 features per image).

Gabor-Transformation [3] is a multi-scale and multi-orientation wavelet transform. The final feature vector of an image consists of the same statistical features like in case of the DT-CWT.

LBP [8] is a texture operator which labels the pixels of an image by thresholding the neighborhood (8 neighbors per pixel, radius = 1) of each pixel and considers the result as a binary number.

Fractal analysis [9] is a scale invariant method which pre-filters an image using the MR8 filterbank and then computes the local fractal dimensions of the (8) filter outputs followed by building models of the image using the Bag of Visual Words approach.

Multiscale Blob Features (MBF) [10] is a scale and rotation invariant method that produces binary images by thresholding the image by means of blurred versions of the image itself and uses a shape descriptor and the number of connected regions (blobs) as features.

3   Experimental Setup and Results

Our 8 image databases are acquired by extracting patches of size 256 × 256 from frames of HD-endoscopic (Pentax HiLINE HD+ 90i Colonoscope) videos using CVC (original, i-Scan modes 1–3) with or without CC. The patches are extracted only from regions having histological findings. Table 1 lists the number of images and patients per class and database.

The different numbers of images (and patients) per database are caused by the different length of video sections with or without CC and with using different (or no) i-Scan modes. It is not possible to extract suitable patches for every video section (the videos are quite often blurry, the distance of the endoscope to the mucosa is too high (no details) or too small (blurry), there is too much endoscope movement (blurry) or no regions of interest are in the endoscope's field of view).

Table 1. Number of images and patients per class with and without CC (staining) and CVC

i-Scan mode	No staining				Staining			
	No CVC	i-Scan 1	i-Scan 2	i-Scan 3	No CVC	i-Scan 1	i-Scan 2	i-Scan 3
Healthy								
Number of images	20	16	15	20	20	28	20	17
Number of patients	13	12	11	13	14	17	16	12
Abnormal								
Number of images	35	34	31	35	32	36	33	33
Number of patients	29	29	26	29	28	28	27	28
Total number of images	55	50	46	55	52	64	53	50

Table 2. Accuarcies with and without CC (staining) and CVC

i-Scan mode	No staining				Staining			
	No CVC	i-Scan 1	i-Scan 2	i-Scan 3	No CVC	i-Scan 1	i-Scan 2	i-Scan 3
SSF	69.6	75.6	77.6	73.2	68.1	69.5	**84.2**	78.4
DT-CWT	**80.1**	78.6	71.9	76.4	67.2	72.7	77.3	69.4
Gabor	67.8	71.1	76.5	61.7	65.2	72.7	73.8	67.3
LBP	67.0	72.9	71.3	65.6	64.2	70.9	74.0	66.0
Fractal analysis	67.5	**80.2**	68.6	68.6	68.9	67.0	66.5	69.8
MBF	67.0	72.9	71.3	65.6	64.2	70.9	74.0	66.0
∅	69.8	**75.2**	72.9	68.5	66.3	70.6	75.0	69.5

For a better comparability of the results, all methods are evaluated using a k-NN classifier. We use this simple classifier since it is adequate for all these methods and because the focus of this paper lies on feature extraction strategies (especially SSF) and not on classification methods.

The results presented in Table 2 are the mean values of the 20 results of the k-NN classifier using Leave-one-patient-out (LOPO) cross validation with the k-values k = 1–20. In that way we avoid the problem of varying results depending on the number of nearest neighbors of the k-NN classifier. The advantage of LOPO compared to leave-one-out cross validation (LOOCV) is the impossibility that the nearest neighbor of an image and the image itself come from the same patient. In this way we avoid overfitting. The row ∅ shows the averaged accuracies over all methods.

As we can see in Table 2 the results of our SSF approach are higher with CVC than without and all in all better with CC than without. The best result is achieved using CC combined with i-Scan mode 2, which is also the best result over all methods. Our SSF approach performs quite competitive compared to the other methods. Only the DT-CWT achieves results comparable to these of the SSF.

Each method achieves its best or worst results at different image enhancement technologies (only SSF and MBF, both using shape features, show similarities). Overall, the best results are achieved using i-Scan modes 1 and 2. CC does not improve the classification rates of most of the methods.

4   Conclusion

With our SSF approach we have shown that shape features of blobs extracted by segmenting an image are particularly suitable for mucosal texture classification.

It also turned out that CVC (especially i-Scan mode 1 and 2) can help to improve classification results, whereas staining doesn't improve the classification results for the automated mucosal texture classification (except for our proposed method SSF using i-Scan mode 2). However, the classification results of the different feature extraction methods are not homogeneous with respect to the 8 image enhancement modes (CVC and CC) and there could be other methods providing contrary results. There is one thing common to all methods, the results using CC alone are below average (considered over all 8 image enhancement modes) for each of the 6 feature extraction methods. These results are even worse than those without using any image enhancement technology (except for the method "Fractal Analysis"). From this point of view we have to state that CC is not making sense for the automated mucosal texture classification using HD-endoscopy, contrary to high-magnification endoscopes. CVC on the other hand does make sense.

Acknowledgments. This work is partially supported by the Austrian Science Fund, TRP Project 206.

References

1. Kiesslich, R.: Advanced imaging in endoscopy. Eur. Gastroenterol. Hepatol. Rev. **5**, 22–25 (2009)
2. Kodashima, S., Fujishiro, M.: Novel image-enhanced endoscopy with i-scan technology. World J. Gastroenterol. **16**, 1043–1049 (2010)
3. Häfner, M., Kwitt, R., Uhl, A., Gangl, A., Wrba, F., Vécsei, A.: Feature-extraction from multi-directional multi-resolution image transformations for the classification of zoom-endoscopy images. Pattern Anal. Appl. **12**, 407–413 (2009)
4. Tamaki, T., Yoshimuta, J., Kawakami, M., Raytchev, B., Kaneda, K., Yoshida, S., Takemura, Y., Onji, K., Miyaki, R., Tanaka, S.: Computer-aided colorectal tumor classification in NBI endoscopy using local features. Med. Image Anal. **17**, 78–100 (2013)
5. Kudo, S.E., Hirota, S., Nakajima, T., Hosobe, S., Kusaka, H., Kobayashi, T., Himori, M., Yagyuu, A.: Colorectal tumours and pit pattern. J. Clin. Pathol. **47**, 880–885 (1994)
6. Xia, G., Delon, J., Gousseau, Y.: Shape-based invariant texture indexing. Int. J. Comput. Vision **88**, 382–403 (2010)
7. Monasse, P., Guichard, F.: Fast computation of a contrast invariant image representation. IEEE Trans. Image Process. **9**, 860–872 (2000)
8. Ojala, T., Pietikäinen, M., Harwood, D.: A comparative study of texture measures with classification based on feature distributions. Pattern Recogn. **29**, 51–59 (1996)
9. Varma, M., Garg, R.: Locally invariant fractal features for statistical texture classification. In: Proceedings of the IEEE International Conference on Computer Vision, Rio de Janeiro, Brazil (2007)
10. Xu, Q., Chen, Y.Q.: Multiscale blob features for gray scale, rotation and spatial scale invariant texture classification. In: Proceedings of 18th International Conference on Pattern Recognition (ICPR), vol. 4, pp. 29–32 (2006)

VISCERAL Session

Multi-structure Atlas-Based Segmentation Using Anatomical Regions of Interest

Óscar Alfonso Jiménez del Toro[1](✉) and Henning Müller[1,2]

[1] University of Applied Sciences Western Switzerland (HES-SO),
Sierre, Switzerland
oscar.jimenez@hevs.ch
[2] University Hospitals and University of Geneva, Geneva, Switzerland

Abstract. The Visceral project organizes a benchmark on multiple anatomical structure segmentation. A training set is provided to the participants that includes a sample of the manual annotations of these structures. To evaluate different segmentation approaches a testing set of volumes must be segmented automatically in a limited period of time. A multi-atlas based segmentation approach is proposed. This technique can be implemented automatically and applied to different anatomical structures with a large enough training set. The addition of a hierarchical local alignment based on anatomical knowledge and local contrast is explained in the approach. An initial experiment to evaluate the impact of using a local alignment and its results show a higher overlap (>9.7 %) of the structures measured with the Jaccard coefficient. The approach is an effective and easy to implement method that adjusts well to the Visceral benchmark.

Keywords: Visceral · Atlas-based segmentation · Image registration

1 Introduction

The Visual Concept Extraction Challenge in Radiology (VISCERAL[1]) organizes two benchmarks on the processing of large-scale 3D radiology images [1]. For Benchmark 1 there is a multi-layered task focusing on the segmentation of 20 anatomical structures (e.g. lungs, kidneys, liver, etc.) in different imaging modalities. A training set of these structures is provided to the participants. It contains a small amount (7 volumes per modality) of the manual annotations of these structures done by radiologists. A testing set also composed of manual annotations will be used to evaluate and compare different automatic approaches currently used in image segmentation and landmark detection. Both Computed Tomography (CT) and Magnetic Resonance (MR) volumes are included in the dataset in contrast- and non contrast-enhanced images. The approaches must be fully automatic and scalable to process large amounts of data.

---

[1] http://www.visceral.eu, as of 14 September 2013.

B. Menze et al. (Eds.): MCV 2013, LNCS 8331, pp. 217–221, 2014.
DOI: 10.1007/978-3-319-05530-5_21, © Springer International Publishing Switzerland 2014

A multi-atlas based segmentation approach is proposed. This technique requires no interaction by the observer and has been evaluated with high accuracy and consistent reproducibility in individual anatomical structures [2,3]. Since multiple structures have to be segmented per volume, a complementary approach using individual local masks as input for the registrations is implemented. We set up an initial experiment using part of the Visceral training set to mesure the impact of adding a local affine alignment based on the volume location of an anatomical structure (i.e. right lung). The results are provided as well as a brief discussion of the current work and future steps.

2   Methods

Image Registration: An atlas in this context includes a patient volume $V_A(x)$ and its label image of the structure created by manual annotation. The query volume $V_Q(x)$ is where the location of a structure is unknown. With image registration the spatial relationship between the target and atlas images is estimated:

$$\hat{\mu} \quad = \quad arg\ \min_{\mu} C(T_\mu; V_Q, V_A), \tag{1}$$

where C is a cost function of the parameterized coordinate transformation T_μ with a transformation parameter vector μ. The label image is transformed using the obtained coordinate transformation. The stochastic gradient descent optimizer [4] with a multi-resolution approach implemented in Elastix [3] is used for the registrations.

In a multi-atlas segmentation approach the labels obtained from the different registered atlases are fused resulting in a single label. The advantage of using many atlases is explained by the removal of local errors if the majority of obtained labels agree on a per-voxel classification [2]. The implementation of a majority voting approach [2] is considered for this approach, but more complex label fusion methods such as STAPLE [5] can also be applied.

Multi-structure segmentation approach: Anatomical variability is a common obstacle for a successful atlas-based segmentation. Since multiple structures are meant to be segmented in the Visceral benchmark 1, the anatomical variability of each structure can influence in the location of the others. Therefore, using anatomical regions of interest (ROI) to guide the registrations for each structure individually are proposed. These local masks are created based on *a priori* knowledge of the anatomical location of the structures involved and its local contrast in each particular modality.

A hierarchical set up is defined starting with the structures that have a higher local contrast in the training set (e.g. lungs). These structures provide the initial alignments and segmentations that will guide the remaining segmentations for the smaller and harder to detect structures. Once the initial structure is segmented a new ROI in the query volume is defined for the following structure and so on. For a start, the method would perform a multi-atlas based segmentation

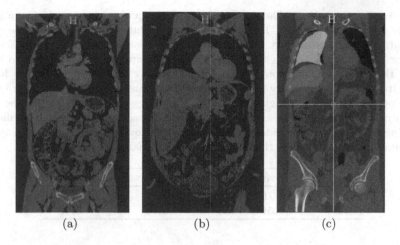

(a)   (b)   (c)

Fig. 1. Anatomical variability. The coronal views of three different volumes (a,b,c) included in the dataset are shown. Images (a) and (b) are coloured in two different regions (blue upper part and red lower part) using half of the slices in the Z direction of the volumes. Image (a) has bigger size lungs than image (b) but a smaller liver. Once both atlases are registered using global affine registration to image (c), image (b) has a better overlap in the right lung (yellow lung in (c)) than patient (a) (orange lung in (c)). If the same output transformation is used for the liver, then patient (a) will probably not have the best segmentation output for the liver, which is limited in its superior anatomical part by the lung (Color figure online)

approach for the lungs, since they have high local contrast and are located in the superior part of the anatomical volumes. We use the upper half of the atlases and query image as the initial mask to guide the registrations. The output segmentation is used to define the ROI for the spleen, which is located below the lung. The mask includes the lower part of the lungs and the upper half of the lower part of the volumes where the spleen should be located. The definite creation of the masks for each modality and each structure is still a work in progress and needs to be defined and evaluated (Fig. 1).

3   Initial Experiments and Results

To measure the impact of an initial local registration against a global alignment an experiment with the manual annotations from the Visceral training set was performed. Seven contrast-enhanced thorax and abdomen CT images included in the Visual Concept Extraction Challenge in Radiology training set (Visceral[2]) were used to evaluate our approach. These CT scans were acquired from patients with malignant lymphoma. They have a field of view from below the skull base to the pelvis. The scans have a resolution of 0.604×0.604 to 0.793×0.793 mm and in-between plane resolution ≥ 3 mm.

---

[2] http://www.visceral.eu, as of 14 September 2013.

Table 1. Global vs. local. The average Jaccard coefficients computed after a single affine registration for all the CT contrast-enhanced volumes are shown. For the global registration no mask was used. For the local registration a mask is created using the superior half of the images in the Z direction. The superior half was used to incorporate the anatomical location of the lungs which are located in the upper half of the anatomical volumes. They are addressed as the first anatomical structure to be segmented because of their high local contrast and bigger size compared to the other structures in the dataset. The average highest and average lowest Jaccards coefficients for a single atlas are also provided. These structures provide the initial alignments and segmentations that will guide the remaining overlap than a global alignment

	Average	Highest	Lowest
Global	0.517 ± 3.6	0.67	0.33
Local	**0.568 ± 3.9**	**0.72**	**0.39**

A leave-one-out cross validation approach was applied to measure the Jaccard coefficient of the right lung manual annotations after only using affine registration. The Jaccard coefficient is a spatial overlap metric where no overlap is equal to 0 and a perfect overlap is equal to 1. We choose the lung because is an organ with high local contrast and it influences the location of many of the structures in the abdomen. In our approach to the Visceral dataset, this organ works as an initial reference for the other structures to be segmented.

We registered the images using only a global affine alligment. Independently, an affine registration using a mask for the superior half of the image in the reference plane includes a priori knowledge of the location the lungs in the volumes. The resulting segmentations of both approaches were compared to the manual annotations of the structure provided in the training set.

Using a mask for the superior part of the volumes gave an overall increase of 9.7 % in the average Jaccard of all the volumes registered. Both the highest score for the best individual atlas and for the worst atlas had an increase in the Jaccard coefficient in all the compared volumes (Table 1).

4   Discussions and Conclusions

The results from our initial experiments support the usage of local masks for structures with high contrast to improve the initial affine registration of individual structures. An initial alligment with a better overlap provides higher certainty to the following non-rigid registration and eventual label fusion. Since affine registrations are less time consuming than non-rigid registrations, they can be added to find these initial ROIs. The ROIs can be redefined for new structures using the transforms provided by the local registrations of the previous structures as input.

Using masks obtained from these initial ROIs forces the atlas segmentations to circumscribe to a particular anatomical area in the query volumes. The definitive hierarchical sequencing of the segmentations and creation of the ROIs for each structure remains undefined. More experiments are needed to asses a hierarchical order for the individual structure segmentations. Still, the method allows for further improvement in each of the registration steps for both the affine and non-rigid registrations. Label fusion is also a part of the method that could be refined once the final registrations are obtained.

In conclusion, these are the initial steps and evaluations for a multi-structure segmentation approach using multi-atlas based segmentation. By adding an anatomical location and image contrast *a priori* knowledge better outcomes are obtained individually for each of the segmented structures.

Acknowledgments. This work was supported by the EU/FP7 through VISCERAL (318068).

References

1. Langs, G., Müller, H., Menze, B.H., Hanbury, A.: VISCERAL: towards large data in medical imaging-challenges and directions. In: Greenspan, H., Müller, H., Syeda-Mahmood, T. (eds.) MCBR-CDS 2012. LNCS, vol. 7723, pp. 92–98. Springer, Heidelberg (2013)
2. Rohlfing, T., Brandt, R., Menzel, R., Maurer, C.R.Jr: Evaluation of atlas selection strategies for atlas-based image segmentation with application to confocal microscopy images of bee brains. Neuroimage **23**(8), 983–994 (1999)
3. Klein, S., Staring, M., Murphy, K., Viergever, M.A., Pluim, J.P.W.: Elastix: a toolbox for intensity-based medical image registration. IEEE Trans. Med. Imaging **29**(1), 196–205 (2010)
4. Klein, S., Pluim, J.P.W., Staring, M., Viergever, M.A.: Adaptive stochastic gradient descent optimisation for image registration. Int. J. Comput. Vis. **81**(3), 227–239 (2009)
5. Warfield, S.K., Zou, K.H., Wells, W.M.: Simultaneous truth and performance level estimation (STAPLE): an algorithm for the validation of image segmentation. IEEE Trans. Med. Imaging **23**(7), 903–921 (2004)

Using Probability Maps for Multi–organ Automatic Segmentation

Ranveer Joyseeree[1,2]($\boxtimes$), Óscar Alfonso Jiménez del Toro[1],
and Henning Müller[1,3]

[1] University of Applied Sciences Western Switzerland (HES-SO), Sierre, Switzerland
ranveer.joyseeree@hevs.ch
[2] Eidgenössische Technische Hochschule (ETH), Zürich, Switzerland
[3] Medical Informatics, University Hospitals and University of Geneva,
Geneva, Switzerland

Abstract. Organ segmentation is a vital task in diagnostic medicine. The ability to perform it automatically can save clinicians time and labor. In this paper, a method to achieve automatic segmentation of organs in three–dimensional (3D), non–annotated, full–body magnetic resonance (MR), and computed tomography (CT) volumes is proposed.

According to the method, training volumes are registered to a chosen reference volume and the registration transform obtained is used to create an overlap volume for each annotated organ in the dataset. A 3D probability map, and its centroid, is derived from that. Afterwards, the reference volume is affinely mapped onto any non–annotated volume and the obtained mapping is applied to the centroid and the organ probability maps.

Region–growing segmentation on the non–annotated volume may then be started using the warped centroid as the seed point and the warped probability map as an aid to the stopping criterion.

Keywords: Medical image processing · Region-growing · Segmentation

1 Introduction

Clinicians have come to rely very heavily on imaging for diagnosis and pre–operative surgical planning. Segmentation is often an essential step in the analysis of patient data. Automatic segmentation can greatly reduce the burden on clinicians who are called upon for manual delineation of organs in full–body scans or other images. They can, thus, save time which they could invest in other aspects of their work in order to provide better care to patients. To achieve this goal, a method to automatically segment the contents of full-body MR/CT scans using probability maps built from training images is proposed in this paper.

Moreover, medical information is being produced and collected at a massive rate and there is a clear need for its efficient processing and storage. This is particularly important in order to effectively exploit the information contained in images gathered for past clinical cases in order to improve diagnosis and

B. Menze et al. (Eds.): MCV 2013, LNCS 8331, pp. 222–228, 2014.
DOI: 10.1007/978-3-319-05530-5_22, © Springer International Publishing Switzerland 2014

surgical planning outcomes. Automating the processing and efficient storage of the huge quantities of data being collected is thus becoming vital. The proposed automatic segmentation technique would help greatly with that. In addition, it will eventually allow for automatic organ classification and, subsequently, effective archiving and storage for later retrieval.

Furthermore, this study is well aligned with the FP7 VISual Concept Extraction challenge in RAdioLogy (VISCERAL) [5] benchmark[1] which involves achieving automatic segmentation of anatomical structures in non–annotated full–body MR/CT volumes. The project also involves the segmentation of a 'surprise' organ. Only training data and no a–priori knowledge can be used for that purpose. A segmentation method that uses the proposed method of using probability maps built from training images would be perfectly suited to achieve it.

2   Methods

A full–body MR or CT volume, labelled as X, is chosen from the database of training acquisitions, Y_1 to Y_N (where N is the size of the database), provided for VISCERAL. Each acquisition has been examined by expert radiologists who have annotated up to 20 different organs and saved each annotation, labelled $A(Y_n,$organ$)$ (where n is the identifier of a particular volume in the database), as a separate volume.

Care is taken such that X is not an outlier in terms of body shape and size. This ensures that the error introduced by affine registration, which will be used in the next step, is kept to a minimum. Figure 1 illustrates the choice of X for this paper and includes an illustrative annotation, $A(X,$liver$)$ in blue.

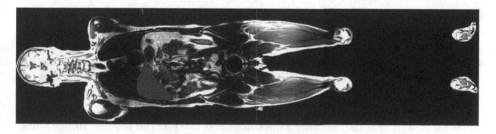

Fig. 1. A full–body MR volume is chosen as X. For illustrative purposes, X is superimposed with the liver annotation: $A(X,$liver$)$ (Color figure online)

2.1   Registration

A training volume, labelled as Y_1, is then registered with X. Y_1 is chosen as the moving volume and X is the fixed volume. An affine transformation [1] is applied during the registration process as it offers a good compromise between

---

[1] VISCERAL benchmark: http://www.visceral.eu/benchmark-1/, 2012. [Online; accessed 31-July-2013].

computation speed and accuracy. The cost metric used is mutual information (MI) [2] as two modalities — MR and CT — may need to be registered together.

To speed up the computation of MI, the implementation by Mattes et al. [6,7] is utilized. To minimize the interpolation errors that necessarily occur during registration while keeping computation time low, B–Spline interpolation [8–10] is carried out. After the successful completion of registration, the linear transform T that maps Y_1 onto X is obtained.

Next, one organ of interest, Z, is picked. The annotation volume, $A(Y_1, Z)$, is then converted into a binary volume before being transformed using T, giving $A^T(Y_1, Z)$. The latter is resampled such that it has the exact volume and voxel dimensions as $A(X, Z)$, which itself has the same mensurations as X.

2.2   Creation of a Probability Distribution Volume

To create a probability distribution volume, the above registration step is carried out for all N available VISCERAL volumes. For each training volume Y_n, a different transformation T and a different warped annotated volume $A^T(Y_n, Z)$ are obtained.

Since $A^T(Y_n, Z)$ for all n have the same volume and voxel sizes as $A(X, Z)$, they may be combined together voxel–wise and then normalized according to Eq. (1) to obtain the probability distribution volume for organ Z: PD_Z.

Please note that $A(X, Z)$ is present in (1) as $A^T(X, Z)$ since X is a member of the set $(Y_1, Y_2, ..., Y_N)$ and $A(X, Z) = A^T(X, Z)$.

$$PD_Z = \frac{1}{N} \sum_{n=1}^{N} A^T(Y_n, Z) \tag{1}$$

2.3   Generation of a Seed Point

The centroid of PD_Z, represented in row vector form as $[x_c\ y_c\ z_c]$, corresponds to the weighted average location of a point that lies within PD_Z. For an MxNxP volume, it can be found using Eq. (2), where $V(x, y, z)$ is the voxel value at coordinates (x, y, z), which is represented as $[x\ y\ z]$ in vector form. For a volume, B, on which the seed point for segmentation has to be found, affine registration between X and B is carried out. This time, X is used as the moving image while B is the fixed volume. The obtained transformation is applied to the volume containing the centroid found above. The location of the warped centroid may now be used as a seed point for segmentation on volume B.

$$[x_c\ y_c\ z_c] = \frac{\sum_{x=1}^{M} \sum_{y=1}^{N} \sum_{z=1}^{P} V(x, y, z) * [x\ y\ z]}{\sum_{x=1}^{M} \sum_{y=1}^{N} \sum_{z=1}^{P} V(x, y, z)} \tag{2}$$

2.4   Region–Growing Algorithm for Segmentation

Current region–growing algorithms only use the properties of voxels in the neighbourhood of the seed point in order to determine if a certain voxel belongs to the organ being segmented or not. In this paper, a method to supplement the conventional voxel-based approach with information contained in the warped probability map is proposed. At the time of writing, investigations to find such a hybrid measure to discriminate between voxels are on-going. Current work is focused on the weeding out of regions of lower probability value from the probability maps in order to determine the effect of doing that on the overlap between the new probability maps and the reference organ annotation.

3   Preliminary Results

For a series of up to 9 MR/CT volumes corresponding to four types of organ annotations: the left lung, the liver, the left kidney, and the urinary bladder, the respective probability distribution volumes are computed. Figure 2a shows the one for the liver, PD_{liver}, in coronal view . The darkest red region indicates a probability of one for a voxel to lie inside the liver and the darkest blue region indicates a probability of zero. The visualisation was generated using 3D Slicer[2] [4].

Figure 2b illustrates the centroid of PD_{liver} as a very dark red point near the centre of the probability distribution. When the same procedure is applied to the right lung, right kidney and the urinary bladder, Figs. 3, 4, 5, 6 are obtained respectively. It may be observed that the seed points are located well within the target organs, implying that the automatic computation of organ seed points yields satisfactory results.

Currently, methods to improve the overlap between the probability maps and the reference annotations are being investigated. It is quantified using Dice's coefficient [3]. Preliminary results of the investigation are displayed in Fig. 7. It is clearly shown in it that the Dice coefficient and, therefore, the overlap between the maps and the reference annotation may be improved by neglecting lower

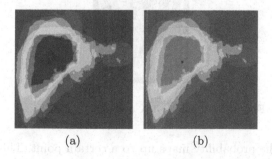

(a)   (b)

Fig. 2. (a) Probability distribution volume of the liver (coronal view). The darkest red region indicates a probability of 1 for a voxel to lie on the liver and the dark blue region indicates a probability of 0; (b) The centroid of the liver is the darkest point in the probability distribution volume (Color figure online).

---

[2] 3D Slicer: http://www.slicer.org, 2013. [Online; accessed 31-July-2013].

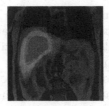

Fig. 3. Dark red seed point on X and PD_{liver} (Color figure online)

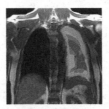

Fig. 4. Seed point on X and PD_{left_lung}

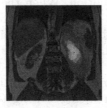

Fig. 5. Seed point on X and PD_{left_kidney}

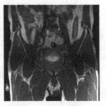

Fig. 6. Seed point on X and $PD_{urinary\_bladder}$

probabilities in the probability maps up to a certain point. This has interesting implications for the use of probability maps as a control for region–growing in segmentation algorithms. It is expected that further investigation into this property of probability maps will be useful in devising an effective stopping criterion.

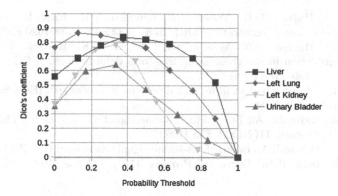

Fig. 7. Evolution in the dice coefficient as the probability threshold is increased. Overlap may be improved by neglecting regions of lower probability up to a certain threshold.

4 Conclusions

This article proposes a very generic, simple, scalable, and easy–to–implement approach to achieve the automatic segmentation of any organ based on annotated 3D training data. Initial results indicate that it is effective in finding satisfactory seed points automatically. Once the measure to discriminate between voxels during region-growing is devised using voxel properties and 3D probability maps, it is expected that fully automatic segmentation will be convincingly achieved.

However, some limitations to the approach are foreseen. Due to the significantly large mismatch between the body–shape, the technique will perform poorly when applied to MR/CT scans of children or people with extreme body shapes such as obese or extremely long persons. Nevertheless, the technique described in this paper is expected to perform well in all other cases. It is also expected that it will achieve the goals of the VISCERAL benchmark and eventually play a significant role in the improvement in the way the ever–increasing mass of collected medical data is processed and stored.

References

1. Berger, M.: Geometry I (Universitext). Springer, Heidelberg (1987)
2. Cover, T.M., Thomas, J.A.: Entropy, Relative Entropy and Mutual Information. Elements of Information Theory, pp. 12–49. Wiley, New York (1991)
3. Dice, L.R.: Measures of the amount of ecologic association between species. Ecology **26**(3), 297–302 (1945)
4. Fedorov, A., Beichel, R., Kalpathy-Cramer, J., Finet, J., Fillion-Robin, J.C., Pujol, S., Bauer, C., Jennings, D., Fennessy, F., Sonka, M., et al.: 3D slicer as an image computing platform for the quantitative imaging network. Magn. Reson. Imaging **30**(9), 1323–1341 (2012)
5. Langs, G., Müller, H., Menze, B.H., Hanbury, A.: Visceral: towards large data in medical imaging – challenges and directions. In: Medical Content-based Retrieval for Clinical Decision Support, MCBR-CDS 2012, October 2012 (2012)

6. Mattes, D., Haynor, D.R., Vesselle, H., Lewellen, T.K., Eubank, W.: Nonrigid multimodality image registration. Med. Imag. **4322**(1), 1609–1620 (2001)
7. Mattes, D., Haynor, D.R., Vesselle, H., Lewellen, T.K., Eubank, W.: PET-CT image registration in the chest using free-form deformations. IEEE Trans. Med. Imag. **22**(1), 120–128 (2003)
8. Unser, M.: Splines: a perfect fit for signal and image processing. IEEE Sig. Process. Mag. **16**(6), 22–38 (1999)
9. Unser, M., Aldroubi, A., Eden, M.: B-spline signal processing: I—Theory. IEEE Trans. Sig. Process. **41**(2), 821–833 (1993)
10. Unser, M., Aldroubi, A., Eden, M.: B-spline signal processing: II—Efficiency design and applications. IEEE Trans. Sig. Process. **41**(2), 834–848 (1993)

Author Index